ADVANCE PRAISE

"This book is an enjoyable, highly readable guide for any woman to learn how to take care of her body–from stress to intuitive eating to honoring her natural cycle as a woman. Dr. Stephanie's fun and engaging style of writing makes this a joy to read, and I know this is going to be life-changing for all women out there on a quest for better health!"

—DR. DALE BREDESEN, MD, *NEW YORK TIMES*
BESTSELLING AUTHOR OF *THE END OF ALZHEIMER'S*

"Dr. Stephanie is starting a movement with this book by reclaiming female wisdom and blending it with modern science. It is truly geek meets magic. It feels like she is your best friend, giving you the lowdown on the subjects you have always wondered about but were too afraid to ask."

—JJ VIRGIN, CELEBRITY NUTRITION AND FITNESS EXPERT
AND FOUR-TIME *NEW YORK TIMES* BESTSELLING AUTHOR OF
BOOKS INCLUDING *THE VIRGIN DIET* AND *SUGAR IMPACT DIET*

"What do you get when you blend modern science, ancient female wisdom, and a dash of humor? You get magic so potent it's hard not to devour each and every page in one sitting. Dr. Stephanie

delivers her geeky wisdom on how to take care of yourself and is someone who gets you when others haven't. If you feel like you've hit a wall in life and are looking for greater energy, a thriving metabolism, and to stop being at war with your body and food, then look no further. This is a book that is about building a strong foundation to thrive and taking radical responsibility that an army of 'Bettys' needs to pave the way for other women to follow. One thing is for sure: you will walk into this book and strut your way back out."

—MELISSA RAMOS, SEXYFOODTHERAPY.COM

"If you want mental resilience, physical resilience, and grit, this is your book. Stress is a global pandemic and the more stressed you are, the less likely you will be able to create a life you love. Dr. Stephanie has written the ultimate guide to help women enjoy both mental and physical strength. This book is a must-read for any woman looking to reclaim their energy and maximize their physical and cognitive potential."

—EMILY FLETCHER, FOUNDER OF ZIVA MEDITATION AND BESTSELLING AUTHOR OF STRESS LESS, ACCOMPLISH MORE

"The Betty Body is a must-read if you're looking for a comprehensive template to learn how to care for your body—from your menstrual cycle to menopause. Dr. Stephanie makes this an entertaining and educational journey to fast track your healing."

—DR. JOLENE BRIGHTEN, BESTSELLING AUTHOR OF BEYOND THE PILL

"The Betty Body is an outstanding job of what happens when you bring science, clinical experience, and a desire to serve women together. This book is a template for any woman to learn how to take care of her body. She goes through all the hormones we evaluate in the DUTCH test and does so in a practical, no-nonsense, best friend dishing on the goods kind of way."

—DR. CARRIE JONES, ND, FABNE, MPH, MEDICAL DIRECTOR
AT PRECISION ANALYTICAL, MAKERS OF THE DUTCH TEST

"This book is valuable as it brings attention to some of the core fundamental principles regarding muscle and protein. Muscle is the Organ of Longevity® and determines everything about the aging process, in particular, especially women during hormonal changes. Dr. Estima nicely ties in her background of muscle, ketogenic nutrition, hormones, and personal perspectives and takes the reader on a journey to empowerment."

—DR. GABRIELLE LYON, DO, FOUNDER OF
MUSCLE-CENTRIC MEDICINE®

"This book is pure magic. This is a practical guide for learning how to take care of yourself from the cells up."

—DR. MARIZA SNYDER, NATIONAL BESTSELLER
OF ESSENTIAL OILS HORMONE SOLUTION

THE BETTY BODY

THE
BETTY
BODY

A GEEKY GODDESS' GUIDE TO INTUITIVE
EATING, BALANCED HORMONES, AND
TRANSFORMATIVE SEX

DR. STEPHANIE ESTIMA

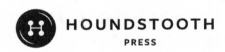

HOUNDSTOOTH
PRESS

THE BETTY BODY
A Geeky Goddess' Guide to Intuitive Eating, Balanced Hormones, and Transformative Sex

ISBN   978-1-5445-1910-4 *Hardcover*
       978-1-5445-1909-8 *Paperback*
       978-1-5445-1908-1 *Ebook*
       978-1-5445-1911-1 *Audiobook*

To Giovanni, who believed in me before I could see it, loved me when I didn't know how to, and who has never been afraid of my geeky magic. Thank you for giving me room to shine.

To my shmoopies, who have taught me more about unconditional love, respect, forgiveness, patience, curiosity, and human potential than I ever could have imagined before having children.

And to you, Betty, for having the courage to pick up and read this book.

CONTENTS

CHAPTER 1

A HEROINE LOST IN THE MODERN WORLD

Something is not right.

And yet, here you are. A free, liberated, intelligent woman. You have access to higher education, food on-demand from your phone, and a place you call home. Baked into your DNA is a deep desire to achieve, be productive, help others, and win. You want excellence in all aspects of your life—from yourself and the environment you inhabit.

You have pursued all the things in life that looked and felt like success—the accolades, the degrees, the home, and the family. To an outsider looking at your life, you are successful.

But something is not right.

You are noticing the things that once brought you joy aren't quite as sparkly. Nothing is shiny anymore. The business, the babies, the bank account: all have come with a cost, and you have paid dearly with your body.

You feel worn down and tired. It feels like you have been gunning your foot down on the pedal for ages without a break. There is an unknown amount of gas left in the tank, and you don't know where the next gas station is for a fill-up, or how much is even left in your tank. What were once subtle changes in your body are now glaringly obvious. Aches and pains linger, sleep is not restful, and you constantly need to caffeinate so you can push through the upcoming hurdles this week. The joy in parenting and being present for your kids has become laborious rather than a labor of love. You are moodier, easier to set off, and even with the sleep you're getting, you feel bagged. In the back of your mind, there is a niggling worry this might be your new normal. The physicians, family members, and other friends you have confided in all seem to agree that this is all a part of "normal aging." They've told you this is the way life goes, but a persistent whisper of intuition tells you that can't be right.

You desire it all: the business, the babies, the bank account, *and* the body. You want your efforts to match your outcomes in *all* areas of your life, especially when it comes to your body and how you feel in your own skin. You have the intuitive prowess to know your body is a temple and is long overdue for a loving restoration. More than anything, you want to feel good in your skin. Goodness knows you have done all the diets and tried all the fads. You've taken all the punitive measures to try and fit into a pair of jeans that are just a squeak too small. You are energetically done with dieting and obsessing about being skinny, and you want to feel like yourself again.

This intuition is the "Betty" that lives within you. She is speaking your truth and wants to come out and play.

Indeed, I did! What is a Betty exactly? A Betty is a fully embodied force of nature. A powerful huntress who is attuned with her body. Her intuition knows what her body needs and how to attend to herself to nourish, not punish. She moves with ease and strength and has discovered the movements her body requires and expects, and she does them. She knows the intricacies of her hormonal milieu, the ebbs and flows of her cycle. She is not afraid of menopause and welcomes it in. She intuitively knows how to eat in a way that is not punitive but a celebration for all that she is. A Betty leans into her desires—what is pleasurable and what marinates her soul in joy. A Betty is sexiness embodied.

And newsflash—you are a Betty. Yes. You. That warrior goddess is already alive within you right now. But she has been buried under the busyness of life. In the relentless sacrifice for achievement, she makes poor food choices and doesn't have enough daily movement. Her voice has been drowned out by the hostile cross-examining lawyer that exists in your mind, constantly telling you that you are not good enough, pretty enough, capable enough, or worthy enough.

But even still, your inner Betty persists and will not be silenced. Your inner knowing is ever-present, waiting patiently and lovingly for you to feed her, move her, love her, and nourish her. Betty is why you picked up this book. She knows this book is going to help you unleash your gifts, rebuild your cellular architecture, and illuminate your self-actualization. You are going to develop a relationship with the most important person in your life—you. And most importantly, you are going to become more of who you *already* are.

When I first launched my podcast, *Better*, I started casually calling fans of the show "Bettys." It was a perfect name that had a cute jingle with the main title—*Better*. The name also fed my vintage heart. And then I happened upon Urban Dictionary's definition of a Betty, and you just about had to scrape my mouth off the floor after reading it.

Urban Dictionary describes a Betty as, "*A modern-day queen, associated with increased levels of self-worth because she continues to create it. She has the power and the agency to be irresistibly sexy and feminine minutes after effortlessly emasculating a mere dozen men with her intellect and ability to deliver. She is educated, deep, witty, and young-hearted. She is naturally beautiful, honest, brave, loyal, and nurturing. She is the whole package: balanced, quirky, open-minded, complex, and flawed. She can be raw in her words and gentle with her touch. She is soulful, connected, and driven. A modern-day triple-threat and go-getter.*"[1]

Accurate and serendipitous, isn't it? I think this sounds just like you.

MY BETTY AWAKENING

For the longest time, I was at war with my body. When my body stepped out of line, it would be punished with excessive cardio, long bouts of hunger, and hateful words. The most hateful of words. Words like worthless, waste of skin, pointless, irrelevant, stupid, weak. Before I woke up to the power of being whole, I was completely divorced from my body. My body was a pain with its pesky menstruation and weight gain where I didn't want it. So, I ignored it as much as I could. In fact, my body was merely a vessel to carry my brain around where it wanted to go. I spent years developing ways to ignore it, and symptoms would be silenced with medication. I would convince myself I had to be productive and that my productivity was somehow a measure of my worthiness. There was always something that "had" to get done that was more important than my workout or taking the time to cook a meal for myself at home.

I was convinced that achievement, success, and the accolades that accompanied them would bring me happiness. I thought, "Hey, if I get on the Dean's list, I might be happy." I thought, "Hey, if I get into one of the top chiropractic schools on the planet, I would be happy. If I open up a clinic and start seeing hundreds of patients, maybe then I would be happy." And in truth, these achievements *were* incredibly satisfying. I worked hard for them and was proud to follow them through to completion. The thing was, the satisfaction I garnished was not what I thought it would be.

I thought these accolades would fill me up, sealing off the gaping holes in how I felt about myself. I thought these things would make me whole and happy and worthy. Instead, these highs were painfully fleeting, leaving me yet again with my feelings of unworthiness. So, I did what any Type A, over-achieving female running away from her feelings does—I set another goal. A new goal I could map out and crush while continuing to ignore my body. And when that goal was achieved, and the dopamine slowly drained from my body, I'd set another goal, hoping this one would be the Band-Aid I was looking for.

And hey, I have a lot of love for myself and the admittedly poor coping mechanisms I had gathered and used back then. I was scared with no guidance and didn't have the tools to deal with my body. It seemed anytime I ventured to sink beneath my throat and check-in, my body scared me! There were so many big, intimidating emotions waiting there to greet me, all unprocessed, raw, and pulsating. It felt like if I sat with them, I would get swallowed up in those emotions like a tidal wave, and I didn't want to hang around long enough to find out whether or not I could survive them. My body and the emotions it contained felt overwhelming, so, with my relatively small tool kit, I decided constant distraction and avoidance with a singular focus on achievement was a better way to go.

I had a new rule: as long as my body responded the way I wanted it to, I would not punish her. I would not spend hours on the cardio machine undoing my inexplicable food binges or beat myself up with hateful words about my willpower.

Food was, as you might have guessed, a big challenge for me, even though I followed my diet with the precision of a neurosurgeon. Foods were measured out on a scale. My weekly breakfast, lunch, and dinner were all prepared and placed in their containers.

Every month, I'd do pretty well until about the third week of my cycle.

Somehow, inexplicably, and without fail, my cravings overpowered me, and I would cave. It was beyond frustrating and demotivating, and I couldn't figure it out. And to be honest, it was embarrassing. Here I was, well known among my peers as an expert in women's health, nutrition, and weight loss, and I felt like my body was constantly failing me. Contrary to what my brain wanted, my body kept craving and demanding food that wasn't in my diet.

My periods, it seemed, were the calculated somatic response

to my punitive measures. My body countered with cramps so severe they required medication. I had hemorrhagic-like flows of blood that would assuredly leak through my pants. Heat and inflammation coursed through my aching joints, angry breasts, and a distended stomach. I would be uncomfortably hot overnight, preventing me from resting. It felt like the ultimate duel. The more I pushed, restricted, and yelled, the worse my periods were.

This was my story for years, until one summer when I went to Italy for a short vacation. After a difficult few years, including a divorce with young children, my clinic burning down, and unrelenting physical fatigue, I decided to finally take a break and go to Europe for a few weeks. It was a chance to finally sleep in, get some sun, and be near the water.

As I began to look forward to this vacation, I realized how much I had run myself into the ground. I was burnt out—physically, emotionally, and cellularly. Looking at all objective measures, my life looked pretty good on paper. I had grown my practice and was being invited to speak on international stages about female health and nutrition. My clinic was successful, my patients were great, but the yearning in my soul to do something else had been weighing heavily on me. This woman was worn out.

I channeled my inner sloth at the beach, sleeping for hours under the sun, and bathing in the salty air. My food consisted of the typical Italian fare: cappuccinos, pasta, and pizza. I did whatever I wanted. I ate when I wanted to, slept until I felt ready to get up, and went for lots of evening walks with the kids.

About halfway through our vacation, I got my period. For some, including myself, this might have been the damper that ruined the whole vacation. Except, for the first time in years, my period was absolutely beautiful. Dare I say, peaceful. She came without cramping, without breasts that felt like they were set on fire, and without any mood swings. She came in like a breeze and left like one. It made absolutely no sense, but I was immediately able to appreciate and experience what normal menstruation felt like.

For the first time in years, I was free from the writhing pain I experienced at the onset of my period. I didn't need a change of clothes on the first day. I was not bloated, and my belly was happy. My mood was happy and energetic. I felt like a goddess. My period just showed up, flowed easily, did her thing, and left. I finally got an A+ on the report card that mattered—the one from my period!

I was finally able to experience great menstruation. It felt like the first time I was attuned to, and in harmony with, my body. But my analytical brain wanted to know: if my body doesn't hurt here in Europe, then what is it about my lifestyle that is causing this?

Initially, I thought my perfect period was probably more about being in Italy than it was about me. I mean, isn't everything better in Italy? The coffee, the food, the air. And surely it had to do with my sleeping and resting on the beach—something I wasn't doing at home. I reasoned that even though my period was good in Italy, it was probably a one-off, and I should prepare for it to return to its normally adversarial nature next month.

But I couldn't get the idea out of my head. If it was so much better on vacation, maybe it was my life back home that needed a makeover. After all, I now had this one instance where my body worked the way it was supposed to. Could I continue this way when I went home? Could I replicate glorious, easy, graceful menstrual cycles, learning how to eat and move as my biology demanded and expected of me?

In the years that followed Italy, I went into deep experimentation. I went back into the lab of clinical practice, testing and retesting protocols on myself and my private clients, and looking for trends and patterns from participants in my online nutrition courses. What emerged is a working body of evidence-based practices that are contained in this book.

I'm happy to report that my menstrual cycles and those of my patients only improved after that summer in Italy. As I continued to test my protocols, I became a Betty in every sense of the word. I lost excess weight effortlessly, got rid of the excess belly fat I'd always held onto, built beautiful strong muscles, got my sleep back on track, and healed my hormone imbalances.

This process and metamorphosis allowed me to fall in love with myself and my rhythms as a woman. It has helped me develop self-agency and an attitude towards personal growth and self-healing that I never thought was possible. I now trust my body. I listen to symptoms as my body's way of communicating with me, and I hold space for my thoughts and feelings.

Best of all, I now *look forward* to my period.

If you had asked me a few years ago what I hated most about myself, along with some physical insecurities, I would have told you I detest my period. And now, it is my favorite thing on the planet. I celebrate its arrival every month.

In my quest to understand how women are uniquely different from men, I have also discovered that the intuitive nature we possess as women has largely been ignored by conventional medicine. Women have classically been viewed as little men or smaller archetypes of men with more hormones. As such, we have been given interventions that work on men but can often have long-term disastrous consequences to our female biology.

To feel like yourself again, it is a necessary rite of passage to understand the ebbs and flows of your hormonal milieu. How to adapt and sync eating, movement, and mindset with your menstrual cycle is something every woman should know. Your hormones are your superpowers, and they have the power to alchemize stubborn weight, eradicate inflammation, and mutate brain fog into ease and grace. Through your cycle, you will discover who you are, how you work, and what you need.

I firmly believe you have the divine capacity to embody what it means to be a Betty, and it will differ slightly for each woman. You just need some tools and tricks to uncover your magic. A Betty acknowledges and accepts all of what exists in the present while simultaneously is excited for what she can create in the future. A Betty knows, on some level, she is important, worthy, and magical.

THE ESTIMA METHOD

In this book, we will unpack the science behind hormones, menstruation, metabolism, and body composition, and I will share my protocols to help you become an expert in yourself. You will quickly observe that while I geek out hard on labs, what must come first is a mastery of the foundational basics. In my experience, starting with optimizing your circadian biology (such as sleep) and menstruation is the first domino in the cascade of health. Morning and evening routines are next, designed to help reduce stress and help you find peace and joy in your day.

Nutrition and movement are the next pieces in your journey. Your diet and your exercise inform your cellular architecture regarding the state of your external environment. They report to your mitochondria on the state of the external world, and your cells respond in kind. Every time you eat and exercise, you are making a short-term investment in how you feel, a medium-term investment in how you look, and a long-term investment in how you perform. These investments are what unleash a Betty.

Accordingly, we will also unpack how to eat, gain muscle mass, lose fat, and support your moods. We will discuss the supplements that are essential for female health, and how to time them appropriately. We'll talk about movement therapy and how to change and alter movement signals based on where you are in your cycle. We'll cover time-tested stress-reduction strategies and effective morning routines, evening routines, and breathwork.

This book will address all aspects of female biology, and I will show you how to nourish yourself and how to move and think according to your female rhythms. This book always aims to answer the following question: What simple strategies can I implement today to help me get better tomorrow? In other words, how can I continue to become more of who I already am and unleash my Betty?

For me, practicing the protocols outlined in this book has changed my period from ghastly to gorgeous. Friends, family members, podcast guests, and even my kids comment on how much calmer, happier, and younger I look. In fact, at a conference a few months ago, one of my long-time friends did not even recognize me when I walked into the room! *That* is the power of Betty. It is the power to own where we are right now and take the necessary steps to move towards where we want to go. This can be done no matter your age, what you have tried in the past, or how many labels you have been given about your health.

I fundamentally believe, with every cell in my body, that we are all meant to experience grace, ease, and joy in our bodies. Let's harness its power and heal ourselves.

CHAPTER 2

STRESSED SPELLED BACKWARDS IS DESSERTS

At some point in my first year of university, I consciously decided to divorce myself from trying to fit in with the social crowds, in part because it was going horribly wrong. I turned my efforts toward drama-free grades. I had a singular goal: get into the best chiropractic school in the country. I studied before and after each class. I wanted to be the best in school. And damnit, I was.

Along with my pristine grades, I gained twenty-five pounds in my first year of university. Forget the freshman fifteen—I'd always been an overachiever, and my weight gain was no different. I'll take 40 percent more weight gain than the average, thank you very much. I began wearing baggy clothes to cover up the weight gain in my hips, and jeans started to collect dust in my closet.

My academic efforts paid off, and I was on the Dean's List. All my professors knew me by my first name. I went to all the open office hours my professors held, read up and knew the lecture topics before they were taught, and created elaborate study notes. I offered my time as a teaching assistant to continue my love of learning and to further entrench myself in my studies.

Yes, I was a super nerd. You'd be hard-pressed to find a student more eager to learn and achieve than me.

The problem was, in order to achieve this amount of academic success, I ignored my body. I ignored all physical signals and pretended I could carry on sitting for hours with little to no movement, eating the cheapest, crappiest food I could find. I wasn't sleeping well, either. Every night, I woke up predictably, between two o'clock and four o'clock in the morning. Of course, this haphazard sleep meant I needed multiple cups of coffee to keep my energy up and my brain awake through the day. I had the coffee run dialed in to the minute. In between classes, I knew I could pop out to the local coffee shop and get my regular two cream, three sugars, and be back for my next class with an extra-large cup of said sugar-coffee in twelve minutes flat. I lived on these sugary drinks along with occasional Frankenfoods from the decrepit campus cafeteria.

As a result of my habits, my food cravings were erratic, my sleep a disaster, and my period was a gong show. My lower back, my knees, my hips—all ached like I was eighty years old leading up to the onset of my period. At the age of nineteen, my knees could predict when it was going to rain. It felt like shrapnel was exploding inside my uterine lining during the first few days of my period. I needed multiple doses of painkillers to get through it.

I viewed my period more like a nuisance rather than a problem worth tending to. I popped the pills and I ignored my aching joints. I put my head down and continued to punch out A's, and instead of resting and recharging on weekends, I volunteered at clinics. I went to the library to study my notes…just one…more…time. I was on a mission, and nothing, especially not my own body, was going to stop me.

The morning after my final exam of my first year, I remember waking up and looking at myself in the mirror. It was officially summer for me, and I barely recognized my reflection. My skin was sallow, and I had large circles under my eyes. My belly was bloated, and I had put on a lot of weight in my belly, bum, and thighs. I looked aged. I looked tired. I looked…sickly.

When did this happen? Baggy jogging pants had helped to hide the changes as they happened because they never got too tight the way jeans did. I had barely noticed my body screaming for my attention. Twenty-five pounds heavier in nine months. Gleep!

It was not so much the weight gain per se that bothered me. It was more so the constant feeling of being hot, inflamed, and tired all over my body. My joints were weary from lugging around weight that did not belong on my frame. I had no energy, and I felt the hunt of chasing grades had run its toll on me.

I was determined to figure out how to get my weight under control that summer. Even in the face of such a drastic weight change, this was only partly motivated by vanity—I was still so insane about forcing myself to get good grades that I reasoned (albeit correctly) being lighter would give me more energy, and therefore a competitive advantage. I thought I'd be sharper and could get even better grades than I did last term! What can I say, with some things I'm a quick study. But the art of loving myself for the sake of loving myself has been a long, slow process!

LEPTIN SAYS PUT THE FORK DOWN

During those summer holidays, I learned about leptin, the hormone that signals you to stop eating.

I had registered to take two more summer classes. (I mean, no surprise there: two months off school? Enjoy the sunshine and relax? No thanks.) When I was sitting in the library one day poring over my student subscription to *PubMed*, I came across a study that examined sex differences for a hormone called 'leptin'.[2] Leptin is the hormone that makes us put the fork down because we are full.

When leptin works normally, the process should look something like this:

Eat Appropriate Amount of Food → Adipose (fat) Tissue Releases Leptin → Brain Picks Up Leptin Signals → You Stop Eating

Leptin is a way for our fat cells to communicate with our brain. And we want our fat cells to talk to our brain constantly so it can report on how much fat we have and whether we need to eat more or less food. It is a beautiful system when all the checks and balances are in order.

For example, when we have a large meal or our fat stores are high, we want our fat cells to tell us to put the fork down so we can use the stored energy we have in our bodies instead of taking in more energy in the form of food. However, with women, we are particularly susceptible to something called "Leptin Resistance." This means that as you gain more fat cells, more leptin circulates in the blood, but your brain becomes numb to the signal. In other words, you don't put the fork down because you don't feel full yet. If your brain is numb to the leptin signal, you'll think you are starving and need food. After all, the brain is no longer receiving reports from fat cells and has no idea what is going on!

Consider the following list of symptoms associated with leptin resistance:

- Inability to lose weight no matter what you do
- Constant cravings, even after eating a meal
- A feeling of always being hungry and having a large appetite despite having excess weight to lose
- Constant fatigue and low energy that is not helped with rest
- Always feeling cold

If you experience two or more of these symptoms, consider that your weight loss challenges and low energy may be, at least partially, due to leptin resistance. That means you need *more* leptin in order to achieve the *same* feelings of fullness.

If we have leptin resistance, we take in excess calories because the leptin signal is not getting through to our brain's center for appetite regulation. The end result is that we eat more calories, put on more weight, and need more leptin to tell us to stop eating.

Think of when you hear a song on the radio for the first time, and you absolutely love it. The first time you hear it, you are singing along, bopping to the music, and letting the rhythm of the music carry you away. You find the song on Spotify and start listening to it on repeat (this isn't just me, right?!). But after the tenth time in a row, maybe you don't have as much enthusiasm for it. By the hundredth time, you are barely paying attention to it, and the effect it once had on you is diminished. Leptin resistance works in a very similar way as the once-favorite song fallen from grace. Initially, it has a big effect, and over time, it diminishes.

There is a tendency for leptin resistance to be specific to females, which is one important difference in body composition between men and women. Basically, the tendency for females to overeat is not because we have less willpower; it's because the signal telling us to stop eating is not getting through effectively. As a result, we can get into a habit of taking in too many calories. This discovery was the first piece of the female puzzle required for part of my healing, and it allowed me to begin forgiving myself and accepting myself as a woman.

Let that sink in for a moment. It is not your willpower that is the issue. It's leptin!

THERE AIN'T NO HOOD LIKE MOTHERHOOD

In addition to our propensity to developing leptin resistance, most women are utterly exhausted from trying to do it all. Data tells us over and over again that women are overworked, under-paid, and undersexed. You might think you should be able to juggle everything and be perfect in every vertical in your life, but life just doesn't work that way. Even if you have the career in place and somehow manage to juggle kids in the mix, you are likely not getting the downtime and playtime your body needs. You're running on an almost empty tank.

I certainly didn't understand all of this back in college, and even many years into private practice with two young children. I was living on my sugar-coffee. I wasn't getting enough nutrient-dense foods. There was not a green vegetable to be found in my diet.

This pattern of a nutrient-poor, caffeine-rich diet is what many women are living today. This is especially true if you are a mother. Moms are chronically tired, sleep-deprived, living on coffee, and leftover scraps of food from their kids' unfinished meals. Three spoonfuls of mac and cheese? Alright, I'll take it. A few straggling crackers my son didn't eat? Bits of their lunch that come home with them in the afternoon? Into my mouth it went. Not to mention there is physical stress that accompanies pregnancy, labor, delivery, breastfeeding, and the years of sleep deprivation that follow. Many of us to do not properly recover.

I would venture to say in my clinical practice that many, if not most, of my female patients neglected to engage in the habits that set them up for success. Not because they didn't want to, but because they simply did not prioritize their health *ahead of others*, including their children. As a case in point, I have never, in all my years of practice, had a *father* call in to reschedule his appointment because his child was sick. It was always the mothers who canceled or rescheduled. As women, we are typically last on our list of people to take care of—that is, if we even make it on the list at all!

Why we feel we must be martyrs and sacrifice ourselves as part of our 'duty' is a separate book entirely. This can stem from observations of women in our families, what cultural norms and dialogue about a woman's place in society are, and what she is told about her worthiness. As a young girl marinates in these norms, they become part of her programming that will follow her to adulthood.

As a woman interested in empowering other women, I continue to observe a deeply entrenched fantasy of women wanting to do it all independently, flawlessly, and with heels on. We are incredibly hard on ourselves, never daring to ask for help for fear of judgment. Our internal voice tells us we *should* be able to juggle the demands from our career, children, and partner, and to always be perfectly put together with a smile. We *should* be able, despite the addition of housework and child-rearing, to drive our careers forward. We *should* always be working out. We *should* always be cooking from scratch. We *should* all over ourselves. It is the self-induced, unrelenting pressure and punitive internal voices that demand a woman must do it alone, without support, without community, and without the ability to ask for help. This needs to change.

National consensus surveys across the United States, Canada, and Britain reveal the same thing: in families where both partners are gainfully employed, women not only put in hours at work, they also spend the most time doing *unpaid* work in the home. Meaning you get home from work, and the lion's share of the cooking, cleaning, laundry, and managing of the kid's schedule is part of your evening.

A recent Canadian study revealed that Canadian women perform 50 percent more of the household duties.[3] In the UK, the number climbs to 60 percent,[4] and an American survey revealed that sex in heterosexual couples and femininity in same-sex couples determined who did the lion's share of the household chores.[5] In other words, according to these studies, if you identify as female in your relationship, you do more of the household chores.

The net effect of this on most women is an overworked, under-rested life, leaving us in a state of chronic low-grade stress, overweight, and hating ourselves. Who in her right mind wants to get her freak on, workout, or take the time to cut up some broccoli for her lunch tomorrow when she is utterly exhausted all the time? The couch and some chips seem like a much more appealing option.

But let's dig a layer deeper. Why do we choose the couch as our solution? The answer lies in our nervous system.

PEDAL TO THE METAL: THE SYMPATHETIC NERVOUS SYSTEM

A part of our nervous system, called the *autonomic nervous system*, is programming that runs largely in the background. It is automatic in nature, and it has two main branches: the sympathetic nervous system and the parasympathetic nervous system.

The sympathetic nervous system is involved in our stress response. It is often nicknamed the "fight, flight, or freeze" system. When there is a stress, either real or perceived, this system kicks into gear. For example, think of a time you had to react quickly and slam on the brakes because someone cut you off on the road, or the instant energy you have when you run after your wild toddler. Your heart rate increases, your blood pressure skyrockets, your breathing increases, your pupils dilate, and your muscles fill with blood, getting ready to react.

This is a state of increased awareness on a target. Whether it be to avoid crashing into the car in front of you or racing to get the toddler before she falls down the stairs, this is a narrowing of your focus and energetic resources. In these cases, you have a singular focus to keep yourself or your child out of danger.

There are three main hormones involved in this sympathetic response: adrenaline, norepinephrine, and cortisol. These are all stimulatory hormones and are involved in focusing your attention and readying your body for the impending threat. They shut off seemingly less important systems like reproduction, digestion, and immune function in favor of awakening and revving up the muscles and cardiovascular system. This is why being in a state of chronic stress shuts down your metabolism. This has a huge impact on your ability to lose weight and might explain why your diet or weight loss in the past was not successful.

Now, before we poo-poo all over our sympathetics, I must also point out that your built-in stress response is one of brilliance, elegance, and efficiency. It will temporarily stop all systems not involved in the stress response to help you immediately deal with the stressor in front of you. I mean, what is the point of digesting your breakfast, fighting off invading bacteria, or worrying about fertility if you are going to die in a car crash in the next twenty seconds?

Your sympathetics will always prioritize survival of the organism over everything else. As such, it is designed to be quick, easy to activate, and short-lived. Now, here is the secret: the fact it is short-lived in nature is the key to its brilliance. Short term, it is a brilliant response. Long term, it kills you. If we are constantly shutting down our reproductive, digestive, and metabolic capacity, this creates a woman who cannot break down and absorb her nutrients properly, who is always getting sick, and has menstruation and fertility issues.

When a woman is activating her stress response every single day on her commute to work, again later that morning with a contemptuous co-worker, and again in the evening with a needy family member, she is effectively shutting down her ability to thrive. She is shutting down her fertility and resilience. The stress response has moved from being a protective one to a destructive one, and the effects are cumulative. The response originally designed to be anti-inflammatory becomes pro-inflammatory when engaged daily.

ONE STRESS TWO STRESS BAD STRESS GOOD STRESS

While the term *stress* is used *ad libitum* in everyday vocabulary, it isn't very descriptive or meaningful. It has become a catch-all phrase for all manner of sins. I could have twenty patients come see me for stress-related issues, and I would likely have twenty different protocols for them.

Think about how absurd (albeit cute) it would be if your child, after falling down and hurting her knee, stood up and asserted how "stressed" she was. Would she be referring to the physical stress of her injured knee? The emotional stress of falling down? The feeling of her heart racing because of the rapidly chang-ing cortisol concentration in her blood? Without inquiring, it would be up for interpretation.

Let's get specific about the different types of "stress" so you can understand how they behave differently in the body. When we think about stress, there are two main categories: eustress and distress. *Eustress* is positive stress. In exchange for short-term inconvenience, this good stress, also referred to as hormetic stress, is one that positively benefits us over the long term. These good stresses may be uncomfortable in the short term, but in the long term, they build cellular grit and resilience. *Cellular grit* is a term I coined, meaning you grow stronger from the stressor in the long run. Like the old adage says, "What doesn't kill you makes you stronger," and eustress makes you stronger.

Tools like exercise and fasting are great examples of eustress. Both temporarily raise inflammation and drive up your sympathetic function (heart rate, blood pressure, etc.), but the net effect over time is development of your cellular grit, or the architecture and resilience of your cells becoming better with time.

Both exercise and fasting have been shown to help us shed weight, generate new mitochondria (your centers for energy production), enhance autophagy (the cleaning up of old or mutated cells), and help the mitochondria we already have to function better.[6]

On the other hand, *distress* is negative stress. Distress, if left unchecked, has deleterious effects on our resilience and cellular grit over time. Examples of distress are bad breakups, falling down, chemical cleaners, processed foods, repeated use of medicines, a soul-sucking job, sitting eight hours in a chair, and being exposed to mold in the home.

Now, if we have been making poor nutrition choices, not exercising enough, and beating ourselves up about it in the process, the end result will be distress. The cells responsible for making our energy, the mitochondria, will be hard-pressed to do their job well. Which, in turn, can lead to hormonal issues.[7]

Within these two main categories, we can further break stress down into three types: physical, chemical, and emotional. Physical distress might entail an acute stress like falling, or a chronic one like sitting for long bouts of time, resulting in compensatory movement patterns or the development of low back pain. Chemical stress might be caused by medications, unknown exposures to toxins like mold, or eating processed foods. Emotional stress could be caused by tension with a family member, an unfulfilling job, and unprocessed hurt and maltreatment from childhood.

These types of stress destroy cellular grit and lower your body's ability to produce energy efficiently over time.[8] Inefficient energy production means we are creating more oxidative byproducts, which age your cells (and your appearance) at an accelerated rate.[9]

Use the following checklist to see if you are overloading your system with distress:

- I need to eat or snack frequently to avoid fatigue or irritation.
- I have salt cravings.
- I have low blood pressure.
- I am wired and tired at night.
- I have difficulty falling asleep and/or I frequently awake during the night.
- I have heart palpitations or my heart pounds for no reason.
- I have multiple food sensitivities.
- I have extra weight on my body, especially around my waist.
- I have a reduced sex drive and libido.
- I experience brain fog, with difficulty concentrating and remembering things.
- I have a lack of energy in the mornings and mid-afternoon.
- My ability to handle stressful situations has lowered over time.

- I am easily startled and/or experience anxiety, panic attacks, or dizziness.
- My ability to tolerate temperature fluctuations has lowered over time.
- I have noticed my capacity for exercise has lowered and exercise now tires me out.

If you experience three or more of the above symptoms, chances are you have been experiencing chronic low-grade stress, which is lowering your body's ability to deal with all stressors—good or bad—with time.

Whether you have one symptom or all of them, these symptoms indicate you are likely burning the candle at both ends. On a cellular level, this means you likely have stress and hormonal imbalances, and there is an underlying inefficiency in producing energy. In other words, you are a woman who is using up her capacity to withstand stressful situations.

THE FEMALE STRESS RESPONSE: TEND AND BEFRIEND

We often hear the classic description of "fight or flight" as the sympathetic nervous system's response to either eustress or distress. A fight response might be visible agitation, yelling, or lashing out. A flight response might be shutting down, withdrawing, or physically leaving the stimulus that is causing the stress.

And yet, this is not always true for women. Women are much less likely to "fight" or "flight" than they are to "tend" and "befriend."[10] We don't start wars, burn things down, or think of world domination. We opt instead to tend to our children, our environment (spring cleaning in the middle of winter anyone?), or reach out to friends to talk it out. There *is* a physiological reason why ladies' night is so important to our health and wellbeing!

I first noticed this "tend" behavior in my Portuguese grandmother. She would rearrange all the furniture in her house, from moving chairs and side tables from one room to another, all the way down to changing where her prized cross and biblical icons were displayed. I later noticed it in myself in school. Around exam time, before I could sit down and study, I *had* to rearrange my closet or a kitchen drawer that was overstuffed. My environment irked me and prevented me from diving into the books if things weren't organized. If I had a big deadline for a presentation, suddenly, my makeup brushes needed a deep cleaning. Before I learned that women react to stress differently, I thought I inherited this odd quirk from my grandmother, but it's a common female response to stress.

Before we give birth, women also engage in tending to our environment. This behavior is referred to as "nesting." Right before the birth of my sons and despite being very pregnant, I was overcome by a desire to rearrange not only my closet and kitchen but to also rewash and fold baby's clothes, vacuum the house, and cook and freeze food for the next few months. This response to distress in women is probably a cry for more *oxytocin*, which is often called our "love and bonding" neurotransmitter. Levels of oxytocin surge when we hug someone, have sex and orgasm with a partner, or breastfeed our children. Oxytocin shunts our stress response and helps us feel joy and happiness.[11]

Betty, here is a moment where I want you to have a gut check. We've been talking about the different types of stress and their effects on our body. I hope you see that chronic distress equates to chronic inflammation in your body. It is equivalent to gunning the accelerator pedal on your car without ever slowing down, regardless of what lies on the road ahead. Eventually, you will run out of gas, damage your engine, or crash.

Put your hand on your belly and ask yourself the following question: What areas of my life cause me consistent and persistent stress? Write or make a mental note of the first few thoughts that come to mind. And for the love of goddess, do not judge yourself. People who are incredibly meaningful to you might cause stress, and that's completely ok. The attempt of being perfect in a marriage, in your role as a parent, or your role as a child can be a catastrophic source of stress. You do not need to be perfect to win, and perfection is an illusion anyway. The point is to begin to check in with your body and listen to what she is telling you without judgment. Acknowledging the truth will set you free.

I OVARY-REACTED: STRESS AND YOUR MENSTRUAL CYCLE

Now, naturally, if your sympathetics are constantly fired up, it is going to affect your most basic functions. It will affect sleeping and waking patterns, and for women, it will affect our menstrual cycles.[12] This means if your cortisol does not follow a normal pattern, starting at a high level in the morning and steadily decreasing throughout the day, it will affect your ability to fall asleep, maintain sleep, and wake up feeling energized. And it will create disturbance in the natural cadence of our cycle.

Women are rhythmic, cyclical creatures of wonder and magic. We want to sleep at about the same time every night, wake at about the same time every morning, and complete one full cycle of menstruation approximately once every twenty-nine days.

Much of this is tied closely with the ebb and flow of our cortisol levels. Normally, cortisol follows a predictable daily rhythm. About twenty to thirty minutes after waking in the morning, our cortisol levels are at their highest. This is referred to as the *cortisol awakening response.*[13] As we move through our day, cortisol decreases so that by evening, when it is time for bed, there is very little cortisol left. No more juice in the cortisol tank, so to speak, allows you to get your beauty sleep. This lowered cortisol, along with some other hormones, allows us to fall easily and seamlessly into sleep.

High-stress hormones make it difficult for your body to wind down and sleep because you have pent-up energy available to fight off the perceived threat. Having constant activation of your sympathetics will affect your sex hormones, and therefore your menstrual cycle. As you will see in the coming chapters, hormones rule metabolism.

YOUR PERIOD: A HORMONAL REPORT CARD

Our hormones are pretty important, as they are powerful molecules that shape our experience in our body. Each time you eat food, there will be a hormonal response. Your hormones make up how quickly you burn calories, how efficiently you make and store energy, and how well you menstruate.

Your menstrual cycle is a great way to see how your hormones are doing each month. Think of your period as your monthly hormonal report card; your menstrual cycle is a vital sign when it comes to understanding your health and well-being.[14] Just like your heart rate, blood pressure, and respiratory rate will tell you a lot about your vitals, the quality of your bleed, and the symptoms you may experience leading up to your period do, too. If you experience cramping, tenderness, bloating, or mood swings, I invite you now to understand that is *not* normal, even though it might be a common occurrence for you. I cannot tell you how many times women brush off their premenstrual symptoms as part of their "normal" monthly cycles.

I once had a woman tell me she has "normal cramps and headaches" every single month around her period. What about cramping or headaches is *normal*?

Now, this thought, of course, is not her fault. Our society has normalized menstrual pain so much that we expect it to be part and parcel of our experience as a woman. Pop a pill and forget about it, like the commercial advert says, right? Wrong. "Normal" and "common" are not equivalents. Normal headaches and normal menstrual pain do not exist. Common headaches and common menstrual pain, yes, but they are not normal by any means.

As you may have already guessed, I'm a word nerd and a stickler for language. I believe language unifies us and defines our experience. If we reach a consensus that premenstrual headaches are *normal*, we will not seek to correct them because the language suggests they are part of our experience as humans. We would not seek to correct something that is normal. If, however, we identify the headache as abnormal despite its common occurrence in the population, we might look deeper into the symptoms with an intention to solve it.

Do you see the difference?

This is important because we tend to shrug off common experiences as "normal" and seek to numb or mute our body's call for assistance rather than find out why it is happening. If you have cramping or a period that is difficult, you are not broken, nor is your body working against you. In fact, it's quite the opposite.

Your body *wants* to be abundantly healthy. I would even go so far as to suggest that your body desires to experience the pleasure, grace, and ease that comes from a hormonal milieu that is harmonious and balanced. This is why she is throwing up a flare in the form of a symptom, because she wants to partner with you and figure out what is wrong. You simply need to be willing to listen and attune to yourself.

The first step in healing is acknowledging where you are right now. That you are probably more tired, overworked, and stressed than you should be. The second step is getting a handle on our sympathetic hormones like cortisol and adrenaline. This is how we can begin to shift our metabolic landscape. This allows us to lose excess weight and to reclaim our energy.

WHY WE CAN'T JUST EAT LESS AND EXERCISE MORE

We have been told ad nauseum that when it comes to weight loss, we need to eat less and exercise more. Hormones don't count. This has been the predominant message for decades, and what a monumental failure it has been. We are more obese than ever before, with chronic illness and lifestyle diseases rising astronomically. The idea that you can tell somebody to eat less and exercise more to lose weight is simply ridiculous. It doesn't work in the vast majority of cases and is particularly untrue with women.

You can't eat less and exercise more indefinitely. You also cannot only restrict carbohydrates and eat all the protein or fat you want and think you'll lose weight. The answer for women, like most things, lies somewhere in the middle. It is nuanced and more complex than overly simplistic models that just count your calories. Anyone who tells you otherwise is sadly misinformed.

The problem is most quick fixes promise the world, and as we attach ourselves to the promise, we reject the risks associated with dangerously low caloric diets, laxative teas, and other snake oil solutions that tout impossible results. We end up feeling it is somehow *our* fault that we couldn't follow a nine-hundred-calorie diet indefinitely or work out for an hour twice daily. The trick to losing weight is playing the long game. There are no quick fixes, and it is consistency over time that reaps results.

So, let's talk about some metabolism basics. These basics will provide the framework to help you understand the principles of weight loss, and in later chapters, we will take this science and apply it to your everyday life.

A basic tenant of metabolism I want you to understand is body fat regulation, which is how our brain and body communicate with each other to determine our weight set point. In other words, what we *want* to eat is governed by and orchestrated by the communication between the body and the brain. If you've ever heard of the term "*set point*," this is what I'm talking about. Set point is a "set" weight we gravitate towards, and it is located in the brain.

The set point, also called the *adipostat*, works the same way as a thermostat in your home. If the temperature of the room gets too hot, the thermostat, which has been set to keep the room a certain temperature, will kick in and begin to cool down the room. If the temperature is too cold, the thermostat will detect it, kick in, and begin to warm up the room.

In humans, the thermostat is an area of the brain called the *hypothalamus*. The hypothalamus, along with some other regions of the brain, plays a role in regulating weight and body fat mass. If you gain weight, your metabolism will typically increase to bring your weight back down to normal, and if you lose too much weight, it will slow your metabolism down to prevent additional weight loss.

Unfortunately, if you have chronic stress, the inflammation it causes will beget hormonal imbalances like leptin resistance and affect sex hormone production. This will cause your body to increase its set point, making you gravitate toward a higher weight. This reality is what makes weight regulation over the long term tricky—it's not just a matter of calories in versus calories out. There are systemic influences that impact our set point!

This is particularly important for us ladies because we are more defensive of our fat stores.[15] We will, by default, keep a little extra padding on us for the monthly energy required to have a menstrual cycle and in case of a pregnancy. With chronic low-grade stress, our set point and our weight will continue to rise over time. Chronic activation of our sympathetic nervous system will over-activate hunger signals and decrease our *basal metabolic rate*, the number of calories we burn simply by being alive. This decrease means when we are sitting and working at our desks, the number of calories we burn naturally will be lower.

So, with chronic stress, even though we might consistently eat the same amount of food, we will gain weight over time. I know, it is so frustrating!

Most women who come to me have been dieting for years. *For decades* in some cases, and quite frankly, they are sick of it. They want to look good in their clothes, look good naked, have limitless energy, and feel good in their skin. I suspect this is the same for you (I mean, you are reading a book written for "Bettys," so something made you pick it up)!

Let's walk through a roadmap to becoming more of who *you already are.* We are going to unlock the bombshell hiding within by getting to the source, healing your metabolism, repairing your hormones, and teaching you how to check in with your body to give yourself what you need.

THE ESTIMA METHOD: SYMPATHETIC DOMINANCE

We may not be able to change the stressors in your life, but we can improve your internal resilience so your *response* to the stressor is in line with your inner Betty.

First, we must focus on your sleep. Glorious, rejuvenating, goddess-given sleep. As we will discuss in Chapter 6, poor sleep is a distress signal, and our nervous system will entrench itself into fight, flight, or freeze.

The second way I like to tackle sympathetic activation is through rituals like breathwork. Emily Fletcher, founder of Ziva Meditation, first introduced to me the concept of the *2x Breath*, and I absolutely love this as a daily practice whenever I am feeling overwhelmed during the day, or as a way to relax at bedtime.

Here's what you do: placing your hands on your belly, you will inhale for two counts, and then exhale for four counts. This way, your exhale is two times longer than your inhale. You can do several cycles of this (personally, I do five minutes of this practice every hour while I work throughout the day), and you may find your extremities getting tingly. You may also feel a bit lightheaded. I love to practice this method along with yogic breathing, or *pranayama*. I find these practices help me dip into my body, get out of my head, and find and release the tension I am experiencing.

Developing a mediation practice is also something I strongly recommend. I try to get in at least one fifteen-minute session in the morning before my workday starts, and if I can, another ten-minute quickie sesh in the mid-afternoon. I usually do this second session around three o'clock in the afternoon, when I find myself listlessly switching between computer tabs, browsing social media, and otherwise inviting in distraction. That's when I know my brain and body need a break!

Another way to bring down your sympathetic tone is through your sense of smell. Olfaction is one of the oldest systems in the body and can be used to bring us into a state of relaxation. The nerves involved in olfaction project right into the brain via the olfactory bulb and go directly to the olfactory cortex. Our sense of smell is so important that it helps us decide our mates and drives other senses like eating. I love to diffuse essential oils like grapefruit, cinnamon, lavender, and rose in my bedroom to help initiate a restful sleep environment.

Lastly, and perhaps most importantly, having lots of sex and orgasms are one of the best ways to clear out the residue of stress in the body.[16] As women, we are the ultimate creators of life, and our womb can be used as the ultimate alchemizer of stress. Get to know yourself (yes, I'm talking about your vulva) and commit to self-pleasure a few times each week. I go over the big "O" extensively in Chapter 6, so skip ahead and maybe take the seven-day orgasm challenge starting today!

I also recommend the following anti-inflammatory supplements to augment the lifestyle interventions mentioned above:

Fish Oil – 3000-3500mg /day in divided doses. Fish oils and the omega 3s they contain are anti-inflammatory agents that help improve fat signaling, and therefore will help leptin signaling.

Curcumin – 1 g/day

Berberine – 1500 mg/day in three divided doses. Berberine helps by increasing your fat-burning capacity, so it is a great supplement to help with overall weight-loss efforts. It does this by improving gut health and insulin resistance and building muscle mass.

THE ESTIMA METHOD: LABS FOR LEPTIN RESISTANCE, STRESS AND INFLAMMATION

Once the foundational basics outlined in this book have been exhausted, it is time to look into fasting leptin levels. While there is no standard or accepted reference range for leptin levels, I aim to get leptin levels under 12 ng/dL.

In addition to leptin, serum uric acid levels will also give you an idea of how well your liver is metabolizing fructose (a type of sugar), or if you are consuming too much of it. If your uric acid levels are greater than 5 mg/dL, you are either having too much fructose, or your liver is sluggish in its metabolism of it.

The last test I like to examine to complete the leptin resistance picture is *reverse T3*. Reverse T3 is the inactive, mirrored form of T3. Reverse T3 is instrumental in keeping the active thyroid hormone, T3, in balance. When we see too much reverse T3, we know it will overly inhibit T3's ability to carry out normal metabolic functions. If leptin levels are rising, so will your reverse T3, both of which will slow down your metabolism. Even though most labs will demark 8 to 25 ng/dL as "normal," my range is much tighter at a cutoff of 15 ng/dL.

I also recommend looking at cortisol levels throughout the day. Blood work is not my favorite way to evaluate cortisol because it's only one reading of total cortisol levels at any one point in time. What we really want to look at is the patterning of free cortisol over the course of the day. This is best done through a salivary collection over a twenty-four-hour period. It's the difference between looking at a picture on your phone and looking at a video. One provides a snapshot, and the other provides more detail and better context. A word of advice, though. In order to get an accurate Cortisol Awakening Response (which is the peak level of cortisol when you first wake up), you must provide the first sample immediately upon waking, and then again about thirty minutes after waking. Upon waking, a normal cortisol range lies somewhere between 2 ng/mL to 4 ng/mL, and the Cortisol Awakening Response should almost double these values, ranging from 3.8 ng/mL to 8 ng/mL. As the rest of the salivary samples continue, we should see a stepwise decline in cortisol levels through the day, making a ski-slope-like appearance when plotted on a graph.

Another lab I examine is high sensitivity C-Reactive Protein (hsCRP). This is a more specific marker than C-reactive protein. It is generally accepted as an indicator of chronic low-grade inflammation, and as a biomarker for atherosclerotic disease risk. Lower risk for hsCRP is typically defined as less than 2.0 mg/L.

Other lab results that should be considered are HbA1C, which is your average amount of blood sugar over the past three months. With HbA1c, I'm willing to accept 4.6 to 5.1 as normal. I love to pair these results with fasting insulin levels (ideally 2–5 mIU/mL, even though standard labs can report as high as 20 mIU/ml), fasting glucose levels (under 90 mg/dL is ideal, even though standard labs will say under 100 mg/dL), as well as post-prandial (after a meal) glucose levels. This is because I want to see how your body responds to glucose because this response is important.

Geek out with me for a moment. Imagine your glucose levels are 85 mg/dL before your meal, and then we measure your glucose again two hours after your meal. You clock in at 120 mg/dL. In my opinion, your blood glucose regulation is great in this scenario. Compare this with someone who has the same pre-meal glucose reading of 85 mg/dL, and two hours later, their blood glucose is still hovering up around 140 mg/dL. This high and prolonged exposure starts to damage nerve cells and the beta cells on the pancreas. I give this example to demonstrate the importance of context. Looking at fasting glucose gives us just a piece of the puzzle. How your glucose is disposed of is another story entirely (more on this geeky magic in Chapter 11).

WHAT YOU CAN DO THIS WEEK

Take stock of all the stresses in your life—the good, the bad, the ugly. Go old school and divide a paper in half. On the right, list all the good stressors you have right now, and on the left, all of the negative ones. Where in your life do you think you might be tipping the scales one way or another? Identify one area in your life where you can begin to reduce chronic stress. Identify some ways you would like to bring in good stressors like the hormetic stressors we discussed earlier in this chapter.

Beginning a new exercise regimen, taking a cold shower, or fasting are all examples of these, and we will discuss them at length in later chapters.

Try breathwork (like the 2x breath) tonight at bedtime and see if you notice a change in your state before falling asleep.

CHAPTER 3

YOUR MENSTRUAL CYCLE. THE LASSO OF TRUTH

"How to Use Your Period to Make a Million Dollars"—this was the talk I gave to the Dovetail Community, a group of high-performing female entrepreneurs doing high-six figures, with many in the seven-figure revenue bracket.

I talked about the geeky magic of your period, how the ebbs and flows can determine which point in your cycle is the best time to give a talk and even negotiate for more money. We discussed the different phases of our menstrual cycle and how to harness it to lose weight and change our body composition. Your period, I explained, is your ultimate superpower.

I only had ninety minutes with the Dovetail ladies, so I started by talking about what a normal menstrual cycle was and how to capitalize and profit from the ebbs and flows of our hormonal landscape. Thinking I could just breeze through this bit and get to the nutrition, I was stopped dead in my tracks. These women—many making over a million dollars a year—were utterly gobsmacked.

"Now it makes sense why I'm so horny at certain times of the month!"

"You mean to tell me this is why I feel like a crazy person right before my period comes?!"

"So, *that's* why I reach for the chocolate and carbs right before my period!"

All I did was use a basic illustration of the menstrual cycle—something these women likely haven't seen since high school—to explain their moods, sleep, energy, and libido. What followed was a two-hour Q&A on periods and the constant hormonal flux we experience as women.

The talk from Dovetail is the basis for this chapter, and in many ways, this entire book. What I failed to realize before giving that lecture is that so many of us are completely divorced from our cycles. We do not pay attention to our rhythms and the cadence of their change. It is in the understanding of the ebbs and flows of our hormonal landscape, the varying daily composition of which makes us uniquely female, that will empower your intuition and give you the ability to take care of your body in a way that aligns with your needs.

In this chapter, you will become your very own period expert—a CPO of sorts—chief period officer. What follows is context, and by the end of this chapter, you'll understand what normal menstruation should look like.[17] We'll go over common hormonal issues and a roadmap to fix it in Chapter 4.

WEEK ONE—THE BLEED WEEK

Your Period. Aunt Flo. The Red Badge of Courage. Moon Time. Crimson Tide. On the Rag. Whatever nickname you choose for this week, your period is the shedding of your endometrial lining. This is your biology saying, "Nope, no pregnancy here, let us scrap this effort and start anew." During this time, you want to pay attention to the quality of your blood flow, as it will give us clues to the balance of your hormones from the past month:

- Are there gobs and gobs of blood in the first few days of your period?
- Do you see lots of clots that are bigger than the size of a quarter?
- What is the color of the blood? Is it dark, bright red, or pink?
- Does it change color throughout the duration of your period? How?
- How long is your period?
- Is your flow of blood heavy? Light? Does your period just start, or are there days of spotting before it fully comes?

The answers to these questions will give us clues about your hormones and where we might place our focus during the next month. For example, if you see gobs of blood and large clots, this may be a sign your estrogen levels might be too high (relative to progesterone) in the second half of your cycle.

During the week of your period, your estrogen and progesterone levels will be low. Actually, most of the hormones related to your menstrual cycle take a little holiday this week. The only worker not on vacation here is FSH, or *follicle-stimulating hormone*.[18]

As the name suggests, FSH is designed to stimulate the follicle.

Think of the follicle as the Chanel bag that encapsulates your precious developing egg inside. Over the next two weeks, FSH will drive the development of the follicle and the egg inside it, with the intent of developing and releasing an egg in the middle of your cycle, somewhere between days twelve and fourteen.

Ovulation, by the way, is the main point of your cycle—to mature and produce a viable egg for fertilization. This is why the first two weeks of your cycle are often called the *Follicular Phase*. It is all about driving follicular maturation.

As you will see in later chapters, this is a great time to dip your toes into new nutritional protocols. For example, if you have been thinking about trying intermittent fasting or engaging in a ketogenic diet, the two weeks of your follicular phase are a great time to experiment.

WEEK TWO—THE WEEK BEFORE OVULATION

Sexy, flirty, extroverted, gorgeous, and horny! Welcome to week two.

Estrogen is making its first and highest rise in your cycle. She is working to plump up our cheeks and lips and making our eyes bigger and brighter. Testosterone is also rising this week, with the reproductive function to drive egg maturation. But a lovely side benefit is it will serve to make us feel flirty, sexy, and horny.[19] Albeit a crude measurement of healthy testosterone levels, one of the easiest ways is noticing a discernable rise in your interest in sex and having lots of orgasms from about day ten of your cycle through day sixteen.

Mother Nature is a wily minx, isn't she? She knows in a few days there will be a viable egg, and as your libido rises, it increases the likelihood you will have sex. And sex increases the chance of sperm being in the drop zone, near the viable egg. Any sperm hanging around for a released egg increases the chances of fertilization. Pair that with the fact that sperm can live up to six days, and this increases the likelihood of pregnancy, whether you want one or not.

So, tread wisely, young padawan. If you are looking to get pregnant, this is the six- or seven-day window for you to have lots and lots of penetrative sex. If you do not want a pregnancy, take precaution here. You are fertile and horny. Contraceptive methods or alternatives to penetration are in order.

At the end of this week, luteinizing hormone (LH), the hormone responsible for helping the follicle release the egg, has its meteoric rise, helping to facilitate ovulation. I think of LH as that awkward uncle who bursts through the front door during a family holiday dinner, hitting you on the back with a, "Hey, girl! How are ya? You look great!" causing you to spit out your food. This is essentially what luteinizing hormone does: it bursts onto the scene, causing the egg to be spit from the follicle. Needless to say, this week ends with an egg being released.

WEEK THREE—THE WEEK AFTER OVULATION

In the first half of the luteal phase (the first week after ovulation—week three), most women can tell there is a subtle, yet palpable, shift. They're not quite as flirty, sexy, or extroverted as they were in week two when testosterone was at its peak. In fact, the hallmark of ovulation, both from a mental and cellular landscape, is a shift inward. In the days immediately after ovulation, there is a sharp decline in testosterone, mimicking levels in week one.

Post-ovulation, it's normal to have a negativity bias in your thinking. What this means is there is a tendency to scrutinize and evaluate the things in life that are meaningful to us, like our relationships and our goals, and where we can improve upon them. This negativity bias is healthy, and a way for us to assess whether or not certain things are still working for us, or if they need tweaking. This doesn't mean that crying, screaming, or having a tantrum is justified here, but you will notice your thinking will zero in on the things you cherish the most, and whether or not things need to change.

This week marks the beginning of the luteal phase, named for the *corpus luteum*, or as I like to call it, the "artist formerly known as the follicle." The corpus luteum will begin to secrete the luteal phase's main hormone, progesterone, in anticipation of pregnancy. Progesterone has a multitude of effects on the brain and body. In particular, she is involved in:

- Inhibiting the pituitary gland's secretions of Follicular Stimulating Hormone and Luteinizing Hormone
- Reducing cervical mucus (lending to dry days post-ovulation)
- Inhibiting ovulation
- Preparing the endometrium for a fertilized egg
- Inhibiting uterine contractions
- Potent protective effects on the brain, spinal cord, and peripheral nervous system
- Enhancing memory
- Slowing down bowel movements
- Promoting water retention

After ovulation, the metabolic landscape becomes dramatically different because now it is all hands on deck to develop the endometrial lining. With this hormonal shift, we will also experience changes in the metabolism of our proteins, fats, vitamins, and circulating antioxidant levels.[20] The last two weeks of our cycle is a time when many women experience a worsening of pre-existing symptoms and conditions. Things like diabetes and inflammatory bowel disease, bloating, poor sleep quality, and premenstrual syndrome (PMS) can all seem worse during this time. We tend to have an increased appetite, with the intensified food cravings and excess caloric intake that are associated with cyclical changes in levels of progesterone and serotonin.

This is worthy of a momentary pause and an opportunity to know yourself a squeak better than you did before you read those last two paragraphs. Put your hand on your belly, take a breath, and recognize that all of this means you are *normal*. You are *supposed* to be hungrier because you are growing an organ. Said another way, Betty, there is nothing wrong with you.

When we are not aware that our caloric needs increase during this time, women who try their very hardest to stick to that *one* way of eating will find it particularly challenging. I know from experience and clinical observation, this is neither practical nor realistic. Any woman will tell you this is the hardest time of the month to stick to that "one way" of eating. And quite frankly, as women, we are not designed to eat the exact same way all throughout the month.

We accumulate shame and guilt about our dietary habits when we assume the reason we cannot control them is because of a lack of willpower. We think there is some mindset work we are not doing as we cave in and fail on a regimented "diet." Yet, the real answer lies in being cognizant of our unique female biology—that we should not and cannot eat one way all month long. To attempt strict adherence (and subsequently beat ourselves up for it) is simply ludicrous. Forgive yourself. Let's just cut some of these toxic energetic cords and let it go, shall we?

In particular, I will offer that it is hard (*nay, Herculean*) to stay very low carb during this time of our cycle. We have different dietary requirements due to the changes in our metabolism. Remember, now your ovaries are busy building up the endometrial lining for a fertilized egg. As such, your metabolic usage of carbohydrates, proteins, and fats will all increase.

WEEK FOUR—THE WEEK BEFORE YOUR PERIOD

Progesterone peaks at around day twenty-one, or on the first day of week four. It's a "peak week" of sorts. It is do or die. Literally. We are either pregnant, or we need to scrap our efforts and start anew next week. Estrogen (or more appropriately, *estradiol*) will also reach its second, albeit lower, and more sustained peak of the month.

Estrogen's role in the luteal phase is to:

- Continue developing the endometrial lining
- Stimulate the fat cells to store more fat (blurg)
- Improve your verbal articulation

A few other notable changes happen in week four:

- We see the biggest drop in serotonin (a hormone involved in happiness)
- Plasma *glutathione* (our master antioxidant in the body that gets rid of free radicals) levels drop

- Vitamin D3 levels drop
- Our levels of circulating B vitamins drop
- Our levels of circulating Magnesium drops

In this week, we will also see decreasing amino acid levels and elevated nitrogen utilization.[21] The decrease in amino acid levels is likely due to progesterone's influence on cell growth and protein biosynthesis required for endometrial thickening.

We also see lipid levels decreasing, which can be due to higher utilization of fat for lipid or steroid synthesis.[22] This is mainly for two reasons: cholesterol and fatty acid utilization. Cholesterol is now being used for progesterone and estrogen synthesis. What this means is you will see cholesterol and HDL reduce in your luteal phase, and your free fatty acids will be used to build out your endometrial lining. In fact, the total phospholipid content of the endometrium increases by 26 percent relative to any other time period!

Another consideration for why we seem so inflamed in the second half of our cycles is the poor or incomplete processing of fatty acids in the mitochondria.

When the mitochondria do not fully oxidize fats, we get by-products called *acylcarnitines*,[23] which are pro-inflammatory. Interestingly, these by-products are often found in people with Type 2 Diabetes and those with insulin resistance.[24] This relates back to the discussion we had around chronic inflammation. If you notice in the week before your period you are particularly susceptible to brain fog and generally feel more inflamed than any other time of the month, this is all the more reason to implement the protocols outlined in this book.

Midway through week four, the corpus luteum (the artist formerly known as the follicle) stops secreting progesterone. This causes a loss of blood and oxygen supply to the endometrium and the blood vessels developing in the endometrium to contract and die. With progesterone's sudden drop, the ischemic tissue, the endometrial shed begins. We get our period.

What I've described is what a normal period should look like. In the next chapter, we will discuss changes to your period, what they mean, and how to heal them.

WHAT YOU CAN DO THIS WEEK

Start tracking your cycle and collect data each month. Download an app that allows you to add in details like mood, cervical mucus, sleep, and details about your period. I personally use *Clue* for my tracking needs, but there are many good ones. You will start to notice times during your cycle when your mood is lower, energy lags, and sleep is disrupted. While there are some general patterns to this, understand you are a unique individual with unique life experiences, genetics, and lifestyle. The best thing you can do is get to know yourself better through your menstrual cycle.

CHAPTER 4

WARNING: DUE TO HORMONES I COULD BURST INTO TEARS OR KILL YOU IN THE NEXT FIVE MINUTES

At this point in your journey to unlocking your Betty, you are better versed in what a normal cycle should look like and why addressing chronic stress is important. Perhaps you are also thinking of how you can improve some parts of your cyclical rhythms and if there are any stressful areas of your life you want to improve upon. Time to grab your detective hat and magnifying glass.

There are several ways, both subjective and objective, to determine what is going on with you. And let's remember that for most women, chronic stress and the resulting inflammation often lead to hormonal imbalance. In fact, I feel we should assume we're chronically stressed until proven otherwise.

For every issue we discuss in this chapter, I will provide my best guidance on testing and what interventions will be of most value. Now, while I like to get my geek on with data, sometimes the simplest interventions are the foundational basics of nutrition, exercise, sunshine, and sleep. For most of the issues presented here, my experience tells me most of the time, for most people, these problems can be completely solved by changing your eating, reducing your stress, and getting more movement.

I know. It is so simple, yet so elegant and powerful. I think most people have such a hard time with it because the assumption is that health should be more complicated. I have had clients come in and have tens of thousands of dollars' worth of testing done. Is this information useful? Of course. But what most women need first, before we are poked, prodded, and examined, is to learn about tuning into ourselves and mastering the foundations of nutrition, stress management, and movement.

Some of the healthiest populations in the world, referred to as The Blue Zones,[25] have minimal access to healthcare, and yet these populations have the highest concentration of centenarians (people who live to be over one hundred years old) and supercentenarians (people who live to be over the age of 110) on the planet. These populations have the rituals and rhythms of eating, fasting, movement, and stress reduction built into their culture, and they practice these rituals together.

Meanwhile, in countries with seemingly advanced medicine, we see some of the most abysmal rates of obesity, mortality, and longevity. While I will run tests, they usually come after helping a woman establish healthy habits that will last a lifetime. It is like the old adage, *"Give a man a fish and you feed him for a day. Teach a man to fish and you feed him for a lifetime."*

The following sections are intended for teaching, married with illumination. They will clue you in as to where your cycle might be going awry. We will also geek out on the lab results I like to see to evaluate a woman's hormonal status.

BUT FIRST, WE PINKY SWEAR

It is important, before we dive in, to manage our expectations and acknowledge that hormones take some time to sort themselves out. Natural, long-lasting healing takes time. Such is the paradox of life—anything worth having takes time, commitment, and a surrender to the monotony of routine. This is no different. In our world of instant gratification, I say, take your sweet damn time. Give yourself the runway, space, and permission to get things right. Imagine you are turning around a cruise liner on your way to a different shore. You wouldn't expect to overcome the inertia and direction instantly, would you? I'd like to invite you to surrender to the idea that if your cycle is gong show, it is going to take some time for it to get better. And you are worth the investment of time.

I will also lovingly point out that hateful words, negative thoughts about your body being broken, and a lack of faith in your body to heal are distress signals and will hinder your progress. You are not broken, Betty. Maybe a squeak bent but definitely not broken. You do not need to punish your body to get what you want. Give yourself all the time and space you need. Assume there will be setbacks. Assume you will fail. It is in the failing that we learn who we are and learn to course correct. Your body is not a machine, healing is not linear, and you need time to sort it all out.

After you have identified where you are, start practicing sacred rituals and rhythms for reducing your stress response. We will discuss them at length and in detail in Chapter 6 and Chapter 7. These are important to nail down as they will help set physical and emotional boundaries around your health through developing and following proper morning and evening routines.

HIGH ESTROGEN: TENDER TATAS AND WILD MOOD SWINGS

Estrogen derangement is generally easier to recognize without testing because we get such good data from our menstrual cycle. Most women with high estrogen begin to notice changes slowly creeping up in their mid-thirties. This is because after the age of thirty-five, progesterone begins to decline. If you recall from Chapter 3, progesterone rises in the luteal phase of our cycle and is the 'pro-pregnancy' hormone. As we move through our late thirties and into our forties, we may begin to notice some of the following symptoms in the last two weeks of our cycles:

- Premenstrual syndrome the week before your period
- Large blood clots during your period
- Irregular menstrual cycles
- Heavy menstrual bleeding
- Carrying extra unwanted weight in lower belly, thighs, and butt
- Vaginal dryness
- Painful intercourse
- Low libido
- Sleep disturbances
- Mood swings
- Anxiousness
- Depression
- Hot flashes

- Night sweats
- Brain fog / foggy thinking
- Endometriosis
- Fibrocystic or tender breasts
- Vasomotor symptoms
- Uterine fibroids

What these symptoms tell us is your estrogen levels, *relative to your progesterone levels*, are potentially too high. This is called *Estrogen Dominance*, because it refers to the relational domination of estrogen to progesterone during the luteal phase of your cycle.

For perimenopausal women (over the age of thirty-five), many experience this as wildly fluctuating, unpredictable symptoms ranging from mood swings to bloating to tender breasts. This is especially true in the first phase of perimenopause, generally defined as age thirty-five to forty-five, when estrogen levels are still high. As we move into our late forties and early fifties, we also see estrogen levels begin to decline, and the symptomatic landscape begins to change again.

I was unknowingly estrogen dominant for years and, not surprisingly, experienced the worst periods with cramps, tender breasts, and weight gain through my belly and hips. I used to blame my weight gain on my genes and heritage, believing those were the main contributing factors to my weight gain. See how women always jump to conclusions about something being wrong with them?

But what does it mean to have heavy menstruation, anyway? If this is something that you have always had, distinguishing between what is common for you and what is normal may be difficult.

Here are general guidelines with some clues that your period flow is too heavy:

- Your period lasts longer than seven days
- You need to change your pad or tampon every hour for three (or more) hours throughout the day
- If you wear a menstrual cup, you need to empty it as frequently as three times daily
- Blood clots are larger than a quarter (although some clotting is normal, the size of the clots should be about the size of a dime)
- Your period stops you from engaging in normal activities for fear you might bleed through, or you are just miserable and want to stay home

HIGH ESTROGEN—WHAT CAUSES IT?

If the symptoms in the section above sound too familiar, let's peel back some of the areas in your life where you may be unintentionally exposing yourself to excess estrogens.

XENOESTROGENS

Xenoestrogens are compounds that act like estrogen but are not.[26] *Xenos* is from the Greek, meaning "foreigner" or "stranger." Xenoestrogens are endocrine disruptors, meaning they will compete for the same receptor sites in the body that estrogen uses and can begin to either activate receptors (like the estrogen receptors in your breasts) or shut them down (like the ones in your bones).[27] This can cause unnecessary growth in your breast tissue or shut down the ability of your bones to remodel themselves, leading to weak, fragile bones. Our bones are constantly remodeling themselves with cells called osteoblasts and osteoclasts. *Osteoblasts* are trophic bone cells, meaning they promote growth, and *osteoclasts* are catabolic bone cells, meaning they break the bone down. Xenoestrogens can shut down osteoblastic activity, leading to bone loss because of unopposed osteoclastic activity.

For women, a big source of xenoestrogens is our makeup! Gah. This was a tough one to swallow after all my years of investing in foundations, moisturizers, eye shadows, lipsticks, and watching YouTube influencers teach me about highlighting and contouring. All I was doing was slathering a toxic chemical soup all over my face. Most commercially available brands touted and promoted by influencers wreak havoc on your estrogen. When I first began to learn about the toxic garbage in makeup (including brain-killing compounds like lead and benzene), I immediately did a cleanup and clean out of my makeup. I have switched to almost all clean beauty products, and always check with the Environmental Working Group (www.ewg.org) before purchasing anything.

Another source of endocrine-disrupting xenoestrogens lies in our home cleaning products and food storage containers. Bisphenol-A (BPA) and phthalates are synthetic molecules used in plastics, canned foods, nail polishes, and home cleaning products.[28] They are toxic to our cells and have been shown to cause hormonal derangement by inhibiting our body's natural immune defense against cancer cells.[29] If you are able, toss all plastic food storage containers and switch to glass or ceramic storage. If you must use plastics for food storage, absolutely do not use them in the microwave. Another tricky plastic is the lid of a to-go coffee cup. When picking up your favorite cup of joe, most coffee houses now have recycled cups, but the lids are still plastic. Sipping hot coffee through a plastic lid is no bueno for our hormones.

In your home, common endocrine disruptors are often hidden in plain sight. Switch out your dryer sheets for wool balls. Use a few drops of essential oil to make your clothes smell heavenly. If you're worried about static, try to hang most clothes to air dry—it saves a small fortune on energy, and you never have to worry about forgetting the clothes in the dryer and having them wrinkled. They hang wrinkle-free until you are ready to put them away! Switch out your cleaning products for vinegar, baking soda, and lemon essential oil. I clean my floors, bathtubs, sinks, and showers with vinegar and a few drops of lemon essential oil.

Here are a few different recipes for using vinegar for cleaning:

Floor Cleaner: Mix a half of a cup (120mL) of vinegar with 1 gallon (3.8L) of water. Add ten to fifteen drops of essential oil of your choice. Wash your floors with a mop and let them air dry. This is good for all floor types.

Toilets, Sinks, Tubs and Showers: Mix equal parts vinegar and water into a spray bottle. Add seven to ten drops essential oil scent of your choice. This mixture can be used all over the kitchen and bathroom countertops, sinks, stovetops, toilets, and almost any surface you can think of. After spraying, wipe off with a towel or a reusable micro cloth.

Glass Cleaner: Measure out 1 cup (240mL) of water, 1 cup (240mL) rubbing alcohol, and 1 tbsp (15mL) of white vinegar. Add one to three drops of essential oil of your choice. Pour mixture into a spray bottle. Spray on windows or glass and wipe off with a towel or reusable micro cloth.

Laundry Detergent: Oh yes. Vinegar can even clean your

clothes. Pour ½ cup (120mL) of white vinegar into the wash instead of the detergent you would normally use. It removes stains, whitens whites, helps dark colors stay dark, and prevents lint and pet hair from clinging to clothes. Again, it also saves a ton on laundry detergent, and not to mention eliminates the plastic bottles it comes in!

ALCOHOL

For ladies with excess estrogen, I am going to make a rather strong statement here, so just remember it is said with love. I do not see any value in consuming alcohol. And yes, that includes wine. Even with the cardiovascular benefits wine is touted for, the amount of resveratrol (the main compound in red wine that confers the heart benefits) you would need to consume to reap that benefit would overrun your liver, stop your body's ability to burn fat, and raise estrogen levels through the roof.[30] I'd rather you take a resveratrol supplement and practice some of the other heart-healthy practices outlined in this book! Alcohol is toxic to the liver, plain and simple. Anytime you drink alcohol, your liver prioritizes processing and getting rid of it over other functions.

I have heard the argument about centenarians consuming a drink or two of wine a day, but I think the confounding variables of sitting with family and bonding with friends can also deliver the supposed benefits of wine.

CONVENTIONAL FOODS

Unfortunately, many of our conventional foods—from conventionally raised animals to produce—are marinated in antibiotics, hormones, glyphosate,[31] pesticides, and herbicides.[32] When we ingest these foods, we acquire this gunk into our cellular matrix. As we consume these endocrine-disrupting foods, we become more inflamed and gain weight. So whenever possible, buy organic meats and vegetables. Bonus points for sourcing from local farmers. I recognize this may not be an option for everyone, but if you are able to just purchase organic meats, this will help reduce exogenous antibiotics and hormone exposure. We will go through exactly how to eat for your hormones, weight loss, and energy in Chapter 8, but the immediate change to make, as much as you are able, is to buy your produce and meats as organic.

POOR LIVER DETOXIFICATION

Now, you may be thinking, what on earth does my liver have to do with my estrogen levels? Well, the liver is the hardest working mama bear you know, but most people are unaware that the liver, through detoxification, works to eliminate hormones like estrogen. In a healthy liver, toxins and hormones slated for elimination are transformed into intermediate substances. After which, these intermediates are made more water soluble so we can excrete them through the urine or bowel. Yep, you pee and poop out your toxins, including hormones your body no longer needs. Estrogen is one of those hormones where we "use it" and then "lose it." Otherwise, it can be reabsorbed, reactivated, and the dominance effect wreaks havoc on your cycle.

For a woman of any age, amping up your liver detoxification capacity is super important. One of the easiest ways to do this is through the consumption of cruciferous vegetables.

THE BRASSICA FAMILY: VEGETABLE ROYALTY

When talking about liver detoxification, we must also pay homage to the royal family of green vegetables, the Brassica family. The Brassica family are the Kardashians of the green vegetables. There are so many to choose from, and all of them are beautiful. It's hard to know which one is your favorite!

These are the most common Brassica vegetables you may recognize:

- Broccoli
- Cauliflower
- Brussels sprouts
- Cabbage
- Turnips/turnip greens
- Collards
- Kale
- Bok Choy

The secret sauce in Brassica vegetables are the life-giving compounds found in them, specifically:

- Indoles
- Sulforaphane
- Isothiocyanates

I call cruciferous vegetables the royal family for good reason. There is a direct link between cruciferous vegetables and a reduction in all causes of death and death from heart disease.[33] In other words, the more you eat this class of vegetables, the better you are protecting yourself from all causes of death, including breast cancer and cardiovascular disease, with cardiovascular disease still being the number one killer of women.

If these things don't get you as jazzed up as they do me, let's just talk vanity. Eating these foods will afford you better skin, hair, and nails, and it upregulates weight loss by increasing something called *lipolysis,* which is the breakdown of fat.[34] These leafy green vegetables rightly own the royal family title. They should be consumed at least once a day, but ideally, you should have them at every meal until you begin to see an improvement in your symptoms.

These and other colorful vegetables are very popular in Mediterranean cuisine. I grew up with my grandmother piling fish and meats over beds of cabbage and collards she grew in her backyard. When you break down the ingredients, the food is so simple. I invite you to think like a Greek woman who makes a skewer of chicken souvlaki over some tomatoes, oregano, and dandelion greens for lunch. Or, think like an Italian woman who might enjoy some branzino (a white fish) with sautéed rapini, garlic, and olive oil. The simpler the foods, and closer to their original form, the better.

LEAKY GUT

Another common issue in women with excess estrogen is a leaky gut. Or, said another way, hyperpermeability of the intestinal wall. This means that the barriers between the intestines and the rest of the body are not as tight as they should be. Normally, there is a structural and functional well-maintained barrier that keeps food in your gut and out of your bloodstream. This barrier can become weakened over time from chronic stress, poor sleep, inflammation, and depression, among many other factors.

While you may not 'feel' like your gut is leaky, some digestive clues that it is might be bloating, gas, stomach cramping after meals, and constipation or diarrhea. Some symptoms may be subtle and not necessarily related to digestion, such as skin issues like acne, hives, eczema, or psoriasis. Other symptoms might include brain fog, hypertension, depression, obesity, difficulty losing weight, Type 2 Diabetes, headaches, mood swings, and joint pain.[35] Although these can be multifactorial and not just from leaky gut, they often occur alongside the digestive troubles I mentioned.

As you will see in Chapter 10, I love to heal the gut with fasting, liquid meals, and resistant starches. Your gut plays a major role in healthy metabolism, as this is one of the places the liver will send deactivated estrogen for elimination. It is also intimately tied to brain health. If we have an inflamed gut, chances are we will also have an inflamed brain.

LOW PROGESTERONE: WHEN YOUR PMS GAME IS STRONG

If you are in your mid-thirties and beyond, you may also be experiencing low progesterone, which can have similar symptoms as excess estrogen. Low progesterone often presents with headaches and migraines, spotting leading up to your period, shorter luteal phase cycles, and low libido. Low progesterone can be summed up by a cluster of symptoms known as premenstrual syndrome. In more extreme cases, it's called premenstrual dysmorphic disorder (PMDD). PMDD is like PMS, except it is debilitating. Some of the more extreme symptoms may include:

- Severe fatigue
- Difficulty concentrating
- Heart palpitations
- Paranoia and issues with self-image

- Coordination difficulties
- Forgetfulness
- Headaches
- Backache
- Muscle spasms, numbness, or tingling in the extremities
- Dizziness
- Fainting
- Vision changes and eye complaints
- Respiratory complaints, such as allergies and infections
- Painful menses
- Bruising easily

Unlike estrogen, there are no foods that directly increase progesterone levels. However, there are foods like brassica vegetables that can help lower estrogen relative to progesterone, and hence, restore balance in your menstrual cycle. We can also consume foods with precursors that will help balance our hormone metabolism. Foods rich in magnesium, B6, and zinc will also help. In Chapter 11, we discuss taking these as supplements and how to cycle them.

THE ESTIMA METHOD: HIGH ESTROGEN AND LOW PROGESTERONE

Take the Estrogen Quiz at www.bettybodybook.com/bonus. Scoring anything over a three is classified as excessive estrogen. The Estima Diet, which I outline in Chapter 8, will help kick start your weight loss and heal your gut. You will repeat The Estima Diet (which is designed in twenty-eight-day cycles) until your Estrogen Quiz score is below three. As you are mastering nutrition, we will also begin to experiment with fasting in Chapter 10, paying particular attention to caloric liquid fasting.

SUPPLEMENTS

For excess estrogen, we want to drive liver detoxification and inactivation of estrogens. In addition to eating cruciferous vegetables, I always take a supplement form of sulforaphanes and Diindolylmethane (DIM) as an insurance policy.

I recommend taking these in the second half of your cycle, daily.

Diindolylmethane (DIM)—minimum of 100 mg daily

Vitex (Chasteberry)—a minimum of 200 mg daily

AVOID XENOESTROGENS

Overhaul your makeup, shampoos, and moisturizers. Buy glass or ceramic containers for food storage and buy organic meat and vegetables whenever you are able.

Follow The Estima Diet outlined in Chapter 8 for weight loss and enhancement of metabolic flexibility. Then, switch over to Keto Cycling outlined in Chapter 9 to play the long game with your cyclical, magical rhythm.

HIGH TESTOSTERONE: ADULT ACNE AND HAIRS ON MY CHINNY CHIN CHIN

Fun fact—testosterone is actually the most abundant sex hormone in women. Shocker, right? We typically ascribe estrogen as the phenotypically female hormone, and yet the frequency with which testosterone issues affect women is just as common, if not more common.

Testosterone is intimately involved in our hormonal balance

and experience as women. It's important for the maintenance and growth of our bones and muscle mass. It regulates body fat, supports a healthy libido, and supports our heart health.

It's important to understand that high testosterone is most often caused by something else. High testosterone can stem from a multitude of places, including insulin resistance, estrogen and progesterone imbalances, lack of exercise, excess weight, leptin resistance, and prolonged stress and cortisol secretion. It is never the testosterone itself but the internal or external environment that drives testosterone dysregulation.

Now when we are trying to understand whether testosterone is high or low, we need to look at both total testosterone and free testosterone.

Total testosterone is all the testosterone you have in your body. Free testosterone is the testosterone that is free or unbound to a compound called Sex Hormone Binding Globulin (SHBG).

Sex Hormone Binding Globulin acts much like a New York taxicab trying to get you to a midtown destination on time. In this example, let's pretend you are testosterone and the cab is SHBG. If you are in New York City and need to get to a meeting, you might jump into a cab (SHBG) to get you there. This way, you get to your destination without stopping at local shops along the way (a definite problem for those of us with a shopping addiction). If you couldn't get a cab, you might walk or take the subway. Because you do not have a direct route to your destination, you now have the opportunity to pop into shops, grab yourself a coffee, and buy whatever treasures you find along your journey. The coffee shops, clothing stores, and wherever else you stop are the equivalent of our cells. When cabs are in low supply (SHBG), it will take you (testosterone) a longer time to get to your destination, and you will exert your influence (in the shops) along the way.

SHBG is strongly influenced by insulin. The higher your insulin levels, the lower your SHBG levels will be. We call this an inverse relationship (as one goes up in concentration, the other goes down). As SHBG decreases, free (or active testosterone) will rise. And here is a clinical gem for you: high insulin can cause *both* high and low testosterone in a woman; it just depends on the patient. Gah. Testosterone is so extra, right?! And as we get older, we have a tendency to become more insulin resistant, and testosterone naturally decreases. Considering that about 50 percent of the population has insulin resistance to some degree, this increases the probability of testosterone derangement as we age.

A woman between the ages of twenty and fifty who is not on oral contraception should have a free testosterone reading of 0.3–0.85 ng/dL. Total testosterone (free and bound) should be between 15–70 ng/dL.

Most women with excess testosterone can also develop Polycystic Ovarian Syndrome, or PCOS. PCOS can have a wide range of undesirable effects from benign chin hairs all the way to heart disease and infertility.[36] As a teenager, excess testosterone might look like acne, facial hair, and irregular periods.[37] This is often when a young woman will be offered hormonal contraception as a symptom reliever. As my colleague Dr. Jolene Brighten outlines in her book, *Beyond the Pill*, oral contraception has a whole host of undesired side effects such as depression, activation of pro-inflammatory pathways, alteration in lipid and cholesterol metabolism, depletion of CoQ10, and infertility.

These risks are often not discussed or even presented as a possibility. Soundbites and oversimplifications such as, "Well, this pill is a low-dose version," prevent the young women and their mothers from making an informed decision. They aren't able to weigh all the risks of this seemingly benign pill.

For a woman with PCOS, the risks associated with taking the pill are amplified because she already has metabolic issues with possible roots in insulin dysregulation, and her cholesterol and lipids are already wonky. With the common "fix" for a cholesterol issue being a statin, this can be potentially disastrous for her as statins are well known to gobble up CoQ10 and B vitamins, which are already low for this woman.

As she grows into her reproductive years, PCOS may show up as infertility, pre-eclampsia, and gestational diabetes.[38] This leaves her primed and vulnerable in menopause for diabetes, heart disease, cancer, and stroke. Yeesh.

And just to nail it into the coffin, PCOS often coincides with obesity. About one in three women who are obese also have PCOS. About one in twenty women who are not classified as obese will also have PCOS. And as you may have guessed, obesity's best friend is insulin dysregulation. If you are overweight, chances are your insulin levels will be chronically higher, which will increase testosterone, perpetuating a vicious cycle.

PCOS DIAGNOSIS: LOOK FOR THE PEARL NECKLACE

There are a few things I consider when looking to see if a woman has PCOS. First, I look for clinical symptoms of excess testosterone-like weight gain (especially through the abdomen and lower tummy area), thinning hair (particularly at the temples, or where she parts her hair), oily skin or acne, and facial hair (particularly in the chin area). Her family history can also provide clues. Are there sisters, mothers, and aunts who have a history of ovulation issues? Frequent miscarriages? Looking at her own cycle, have any cycles been longer than thirty-five days? Is there a current or previous history of periods being missed altogether?

Then we move into lab work. I would be looking for high free and/or total testosterone from blood work and/or urine samples. As I mentioned before, getting bloodwork is like taking a picture on your phone and urine testing is like a video—both give us valuable information, but the urine sample will clue us into how the testosterone is being metabolized and broken down. I would also look at fasted glucose and post-prandial glucose challenge tests as described in the previous section. If we can time it right, we go into the lab to look for an LH surge right around ovulation (day twelve to fourteen of the cycle), and then again at day twenty-one of the cycle to look for a rise in progesterone.

Lastly, and pulling it all together, we can look at physical evidence of the cysts. This is confirmed by ultrasound of the ovaries. *Pearl necklace sign* is the name for the finding on an ultrasound that shows a cluster of 8 mm cysts on the ovaries, with an average of twelve cysts per ovary. These are consistent with the Androgen Excess and PCOS Society criteria for diagnosis of Polycystic Ovarian Syndrome.[39]

I have provided a testosterone quiz at www.bettybodybook.com/bonus to subjectively see if the symptoms you are experiencing are consistent with those of high testosterone. Now this quiz is not diagnostic but rather an initial inquiry as to whether high testosterone might be at the root of your period problems. But this is a great place to start—it takes most women with PCOS an average of seven years to get diagnosed, which is a hell of a long time to wait for an answer!

HIGH TESTOSTERONE: THE ESTIMA METHOD

The good news is that manipulating variables such as exercise, nutrition, fasting, and stress management can have profound effects on bringing elevated testosterone levels back to normal.

Women with high levels of testosterone due to insulin resistance respond well by adding in resistance and high-intensity interval training, lowering carbohydrate intake, and engaging in fasting.[40] We will cover this in great detail in Chapters 8, 9, and 10. As it relates to body composition, the key is to build up your lean muscle mass. This will help to dispose of glucose more effectively (muscle likes to gobble up glucose for its own use), thereby helping to lower the insulinergic response to blood glucose. In other words, the more muscle you have, the more it acts like a glucose sink, draining excess sugar out of the blood and into the muscles. This will help to lower inflammation and rev up your metabolism to reduce excess weight. Muscles are our goddess-given solution to a myriad of sins.

In The Estima Diet outlined in Chapter 8, you will eat oodles of green leafy vegetables, which are bursting with fiber, zinc, and other phytonutrients. You will consume lots of heart-healthy fats like avocados, nuts, and seeds, and get rid of all processed sugar.

Pay particular attention to the water fasting in Chapter 10. At the end of the twelve-week fasting program, aiming for one to two days per week of twenty-four-hour water fasting is ideal. You might also consider a longer water fast the week of your period.

Use stress management techniques like the ones outlined in Chapters 6 and 7, and make sure you sleep at least eight hours per night.

> Supplements I use to help correct insulin dysregulation are Berberine (1500-2000mg/day in three divided doses), Alpha Lipoic Acid (1000 mg/day), and Omega 3s (2g/day in two divided doses).

LOW TESTOSTERONE: PAINFUL SEX, BACK FAT, AND HAIR LOSS. F'N GREAT.

Finding hormonal balance often reminds me of the children's fable, *Goldilocks and the Three Bears*. When it comes to hormones, they have to be *juuust right*, and we see this with testosterone. As I mentioned in the previous section, we definitely need testosterone to drive up our muscle mass, bone density, and libido, but having too little of it has its own particular set of problems. This is true as it relates to the impact testosterone has on the musculature of the vagina and the pelvic floor. Low testosterone is associated with vaginal wall atrophy. The vagina and pelvic floor are composed of muscle, and when we orgasm, these muscles contract in a rhythmic fashion to facilitate moving the sperm up towards the cervix. If these muscles atrophy, you might experience numbness or lack of sensation in the vagina during sex, poor lubrication or the feeling of being "dry," and painful sex. In the extreme, you may also experience anorgasmia because the pelvic floor muscles that facilitate these rhythmic contractions simply cannot contract.

A yellow flag signaling possible low testosterone goes up when a woman tells me that the physical activities she once enjoyed are now leaving her spent or exhausted for the rest of the day. She will often describe fatigue that is unrelieved by sleep, even when it is supplemented with naps throughout the day. That is when I add low testosterone as a possibility to my list of differentials. Another flag goes up when she tells me her libido stays the same all month long. Normally, around day ten of your cycle, you should notice an uptick in your interest in sex. If not, it may be an indicator, albeit a crude one, of decreased testosterone.

Hair loss is also common with low testosterone, as is weight gain around the abdomen. As the quantity of the hair on our head decreases, it will also tend to lose its glossy, shiny quality. A woman will often tell me she needs to wrap the band for her ponytail or bun around her hair more times than she used to, or that she has noticed a thinning out of her pubic, underarm, or leg hair.

LOW TESTOSTERONE—CAUSES

There is a myriad of reasons why your testosterone might be low, with the most common one being aging. As we age, there is a natural drop in the androgens we produce. This is why building muscle is so incredibly vital for you, which is outlined in Chapter 11. Other reasons range from oophorectomy (surgical removal of the ovaries), chemical oophorectomy (from chemotherapy or radiation therapy), the pill or any form of estrogen therapy, and extreme dieting. This is why I rally so hard against caloric restriction for women. It cannot be sustained over the long term and has devastating consequences for testosterone levels in women.

It's tricky to diagnose low testosterone because it often presents like other common issues. If a woman comes to me and says, "Hey, Doc, I've been gaining weight, I'm exhausted, I'm always cold, and I can't sleep," one must tread carefully. These are *the exact symptoms* of an underactive thyroid, iron deficiency anemia, depression, and many autoimmune conditions. Testosterone is also tricky because it is difficult to measure. The amount of circulating testosterone is not the same as the active amount inside the cells.

To make things even more confusing, a woman's results can vary depending on when the test is taken, both in her cycle and the time of day. So, if you are having labs done, the collection should be taken in the morning, when your testosterone levels are at their highest, ideally eight to sixteen days after the start of your period.

LOW TESTOSTERONE: THE ESTIMA METHOD

The good news with low testosterone is that foundational basics like diet and exercise can strongly influence and improve it. Lucky for you, we are going on a geeky magic carpet ride in this book on these very subjects.

In terms of nutrition, the first phase of The Estima Diet will be particularly useful for you to help lower insulin secretion and get more testosterone into the cells to do its work. The second part of our nutrition journey will look at cycling high protein, which will help you drive muscle protein synthesis and testosterone levels. In terms of exercise, leaning into resistance training will drive more muscle mass, and more testosterone. We discuss this at length in Chapter 9 when we discuss cycling protein through the month.

Paying particular attention to your stress levels and sleep quality will also help level out low testosterone. Many women I have treated with low testosterone have extraordinary amounts of anxiety and depression, and very poor quality of sleep. Setting up your morning and evening routines to start and end your days right will be enormously helpful.

Lastly, building muscle will help to naturally elevate your testosterone levels.[41] The more muscle mass we have, the more testosterone we have. Coupling nutrition with exercise therapy (in Chapters 8, 9, and 11, respectively) will be the best natural tool you have to improve testosterone.

WHAT YOU CAN DO THIS WEEK

Start tracking your foods. Before you get to the nutritional and training sections in this book, it will be super valuable for you to quantify your eating habits throughout your cycle. You will begin to notice when you feel energetically low, when you reach for certain foods, the timing of your meals, and the composition of your diet. While most of us visually estimate and guess how much food we eat without tracking, most people underreport caloric intake anywhere from 30–50 percent. I use a free app called Carb Manager, which allows me to set the number of calories and ratios of foods I want to consume for the day.

Take the hormone quizzes at www.bettybodybook.com/bonus as a baseline measurement. It is so easy for us to forget where we start, making it nearly impossible to evaluate how much progress we've made! Remember what you looked and felt like six months ago? Yea, me neither.

CHAPTER 5

I'M STILL HOT. IT JUST COMES IN FLASHES NOW. PERIMENOPAUSE, MENOPAUSE, AND LOW ESTROGEN

"I don't intend to grow old gracefully, I intend to fight it every step of the way."

—OIL OF OLAY AD SLOGAN

When we listen to marketing dogma like this, which is intended to sell you toxic face cream, it's no wonder we fear aging. As a culture, I believe we are psychologically primed to be afraid of menopause. Women are called spinsters, hags, crones, frump, matronly, old maids. And where are the sexy sixty-year-old women in movies? We hardly see menopausal women play roles in movies who own their sexiness, have lots of great sex, believe in themselves, love their bodies, and wear clothes that make them feel good.

However, I believe the landscape is changing for what we expect of women in this era. We are seeing celebrities redefine what it means to be a woman at fifty, sixty, and beyond. Menopause does not need to be a time where you lose your femininity, sexuality, drive, and personality. It is a time where we can, with absolute grace and ease, get comfortable in our skin, with who we are, what we have experienced, and love our bodies.

And just think of the freedom you'll have in menopause. The energy you used every month to develop a womb can now be used for other pursuits you love. It is just a matter of harnessing this power effectively.

Perimenopause is not so much a diagnosis as it is a spectrum. There is no defined beginning, and the symptoms vary widely from woman to woman. Most women are shocked to learn that sex hormones start to decline in our mid-thirties! It's true, and it's nothing to be alarmed by. At about the age of thirty-five, we start to see progesterone, estrogen, and testosterone begin to decline. In the previous chapter, we talked about estrogen dominance and low progesterone. If you are in your mid- to late thirties and find your symptoms of estrogen dominance worsening, this is one of the first signs that your sex hormones are declining.

Some women can breeze through menopause like it is any other event on their calendar. Other women...ooofala. It is a nightmare! Everything from excessive fatigue, concentration problems, unexplained weight gain, brain fog, feeling inflamed, gut issues (bloating, gassy after meals), night sweats, memory changes (why did I walk into this room again?), waning interest in sex, hot flashes, and night sweats.

HOW DO I KNOW IF I'M IN PERIMENOPAUSE?

There are some clues to help you identify if you are in perimenopause. In the beginning, women notice their period comes a day or two ahead of when it was supposed to come. Shorter cycle length is a very common sign of early perimenopause. So, if you are used to getting your period every twenty-eight days, you might notice it is starting to come a day or two earlier each month, and it might be accompanied by some spotting right before it starts.

Then, as you progress to later in the process, it is likely the opposite will happen—instead of coming closer together, your period cycle starts to lengthen. I will often have women report skipping a period one month, only to have it return the following month with a super heavy flow. Over time, your cycle will continue to lengthen. Instead of skipping one month, your period might go missing in action for a few months, and then return.

The journey to menopause can be unpredictable, and sometimes frightening. I have had women report that they skip three months, and then subsequently bleed for weeks, which can be very scary. To make matters worse, the technical definition of menopause is only given once you have not had your period for twelve consecutive months. This can be confusing for a woman who has not had her period for three months. She has to wait another nine months for the label of menopause because by its nature, it is a retroactive definition.

If I may, I'd like to introduce a radical thought. I would love for you to acknowledge that your body is not working against you, despite these erratic times. She is preparing you for the next stage of your life. By leaning in, listening to your body, and using the frameworks in this book, you can trust yourself and the process.

ESTROGEN CHANGES IN PERIMENOPAUSE

As we discussed in the previous chapter, early menopause is often characterized as estrogen dominance relative to progesterone. If you remember from Chapter 3, in the second half of your cycle, progesterone is the star of the show in your luteal phase. She peaks at the beginning of week four of your cycle. In our early forties, as progesterone drops, we may see her sister, estrogen, unintentionally stealing the show during this time. Hence the term estrogen dominance.

However, as we move toward menopause, we begin to see estrogen levels decline.

Declining estrogen can be a murky time because this is the hormone that defines us as feminine. It drives up our cheekbones, plumps our skin, glosses up our hair, and contributes to the maintenance of our female reproductive organs. In addition to testosterone, estrogens are involved in the maintenance of our vaginal wall, pelvic floor, and our vulva tissues.

In the same way normal levels of progesterone stimulate appetite, low estrogen has the same effect.[42] Women in their late 40s often complain of wanting to lose weight, with impossible cravings that persist no matter what they tried in the past, even if it was a form of the ketogenic diet.

This is why it's important to create a female-centric ketogenic diet that spans across your life. For women with low estrogen, resistant starches may be just the trick to help with persistent cravings that lead to weight gain. As the name suggests, resistant starches resist digestion, much like insoluble fiber. What happens is these resistant starches will pass through the intestinal tract, and once they arrive in the large intestine, they serve as food for the microbiome there. Regular resistant starch consumption has been associated with an improvement in insulin sensitivity, fat burning, and increasing diversity in the gut microbiome.[43] This is the key to the sustainability of this diet.

Around week three or four on a ketogenic diet, most women complain of strong cravings that no amount of fat can quell. What drives that insatiable craving is the starving microbiome. Adding in resistant starches will not only feed these little critters, but they reward you by producing butyrate, a short-chain fatty acid. Butyrate has been shown to help with sleep, repair the lining of the gut, and deepen your ketogenic state.

Examples of resistant starches are green banana flour, green plantain flour, raw potato starch, cold rice, cold potatoes, and green bananas. The way I advise you to consume your resistant starches is to take 1 tsp per day, either in water or in a smoothie. I strongly recommend starting off with green banana flour, green plantain flour, or raw potato starch to begin, because the amount of resistant starches is known. These are easily sourced at online retailers or at natural food grocers. When we use cold rice or cold potatoes, we don't know the exact amount of resistant starches contained within them (although the more you reheat and cool them, the higher the resistant starch percentage).

So, if you are a woman in her late forties with insatiable cravings and stubborn weight gain that just won't quit, the addition of resistant starches in The Estima Diet will help immensely to curb the cravings.

The other consideration for women in their forties with low estrogen is bone health. Bones, in all their glory, not only act as scaffolding for your entire frame. It's also been suggested they play a role in the acute stress response.[44] They are constantly remolding their architecture, and we have an entirely new skeleton approximately every two to three years. This happens because of the dance between osteoblasts and osteoclasts.

If you recall from the previous chapter, we discussed the impact xenoestrogens have on the balance between these two types of bone cells. Since estrogen is a hormone that stimulates growth, it affects these two bone cells. As estrogen levels drop, we begin to see an increase in osteoclastic activity *relative* to osteoblastic activity. Left unchecked, at best, it means osteopenia, and at worst, osteoporosis. Bones with osteoporosis look like Swiss cheese on a molecular level. They are pock-marked, brittle, and susceptible to fractures. This is why resistance training is so important! Muscles and bones are intimately connected. As we increase our muscle mass, we also increase our bone density.

LOW ESTROGEN—CAUSES

As we have been discussing, our estrogen levels naturally decline with age, particularly in the latter half of our forties. There are some other ways we prematurely lower estrogen levels, and they are eerily similar to some of the causes of low testosterone. First and foremost, extreme exercise or extreme caloric restriction resulting in low body-fat levels can put estrogen levels in the tank and leave you without a period.

I can attest to this personally, and I experienced this when I decided to compete in a figure competition, as well as when I tried to fast for too long. The figure competition was always on my bucket list, and for the most part the training and eating was incredibly healthy. That is, of course, until I got to peak week. "Peak week" is a week from hell where you drink an absurd amount of water, and then you abstain from it right before the show so you can get rid of any subcutaneous water in the appearance of muscles. This is the time-tested technique that many fitness models use right before a photoshoot to get rid of excess water for a very short period of time. There is also severe caloric restriction and long hours of training that accompanied the water debauchery. While I did well in the competition (I placed third overall), it wreaked havoc on my menstrual cycle for the next three months. I had hot flashes. I was depressed, had zero energy, and had ridiculous cravings. It made me realize it was the first and last competition I would ever do.

Another commonality low estrogen has with low testosterone is atrophy to the vaginal wall and pelvic floor. This can include symptoms of vaginal dryness, painful sex, a reduced interest in sex, and vaginal wall atrophy. Fatigue and low energy that are unrelieved by sleep or napping is another clue.

To determine if you have low estrogen, you will want to look at serum estradiol. Estradiol is the most potent and abundant estrogen and can be used as a proxy for total estrogen in the body. I want to see serum progesterone and estradiol to understand the relative amounts of these sister hormones in comparison to each other. I also want to look at Sex Hormone Binding Globulin (SHBG). It's helpful to check this when all your other labs look normal, but you are experiencing the symptoms we described above.

Knowing where you are in your cycle, as we described in Chapter 3, is incredibly important. In the follicular phase (the first two weeks of your cycle), estrogen is very low in week one and reaches an astronomical peak in week two. Estradiol levels move anywhere from 20 pg/mL to 200 pg/mL. And even if you fall within this relatively large bracket, you might be a low normal, or in a lower percentile of normal, which may be driving these symptoms. I define low estrogen as less than 15 pg/mL.

THE ESTIMA DIET FOR PERIMENOPAUSE

In terms of hormones, the biggest focus for women in early-stage perimenopause is to attempt to get the progesterone-estrogen balance back. This means decreasing excess estrogen in the second half of your cycle. When we see low estrogens in late perimenopause, we need to fortify our adrenal glands, which will be one of the main sources of estrogen production after the ovaries retire.

And as much as we are going to nerd out on nutrition and fitness, you cannot eat your way out of a stressed mind. It is absolutely essential to look at your mental health and wellbeing to reduce your cortisol and stress levels. This includes optimizing your circadian biology and getting your morning and evening routines dialed in, even if they are only five minutes (as mine often are).

The second step is to reduce your perceived stress and your response to it. Remember in Chapter 3 we talked about the harrowing consequences of too much stress, its effect on cortisol, mitochondrial health, and your energy? Remember, a stressor (like a child, a boss, or a partner) is only a stressor once you label and react to it as one. Being able to remain in a state of ease and grace is what we are moving towards. This is important as our stress levels will negatively affect our insulin levels. If you recall, insulin is the hormone that brings glucose into the cell. When there is constant cortisol and other stress hormones hanging out, they will prevent insulin from doing its job properly.

It has been my observation that insulin, a metabolic hormone, is a driving contributor to the symptoms women experience in perimenopause. While we tend to focus solely on estrogen, progesterone, and testosterone, which are all super important, I think insulin is also a main player in symptom management.

It is true that as we age, we generally become more insulin resistant. There are a few ways to help determine the extent to which this is happening.

First, take your waist to hip ratio. You want to measure your natural waist. This is usually around the navel, or if your navel has migrated south after childbirth, it is the narrowest part of your waist. For your hip measurement, measure around the widest part of your hips. Once you have these two measurements, divide your waist number by your hip number. This ratio should be less than 0.8. I like this as a general measurement because it takes the focus off weight and places it on your proportions. Personally, I think we are too obsessed as a culture with weight, which fails to account for body composition.

If you are a data nerd (hello, my geeky magic friend), you can also monitor your fasting blood glucose. I like to see numbers under 90 mg/dL, ideally between 80–85 mg/dL.

From a nutritional perspective, following The Estima Diet outlined in Chapter 8 will be a therapeutic intervention to lower insulin and help kick-start weight loss. This excess weight is usually a consequence of going through perimenopause and menopause. This protocol will also help reduce some of the common symptoms women experience from either low estrogen, excess insulin, or excess gluten. In Chapter 11, we will also discuss how to begin to build lean muscle mass. This is so important for women in perimenopause and menopause because the more muscle mass you have, the better glucose disposal agent you are. Meaning, you can dump glucose from the blood into muscle.

But wait, there's more!

The more muscle mass you have, the more testosterone you will have, and many women who experience low testosterone or low estrogen experience some of the common complaints in menopause like low libido, painful sex, poor vaginal lubrication, and difficulty having orgasms. This is something women are embarrassed to talk about, and some may not even realize it's happening.

Soooo…needless to say, boatloads of sex and orgasms are important for improving the estrogen balance. Doctors' orders! From an evolutionary perspective, the more sex and orgasms you have, the more reproductively useful you appear to be. In Chapter 6, we will do a deep dive into sex and orgasms, but the takeaway here is *orgasm*. And do it often. Orgasms and pleasure are not only your birthright, but they will help contribute to happy hormones.

I also love to incorporate supplements like black cohosh (100 mg daily in divided doses), and Vitex Agnus-Castus (200 mg in divided doses throughout the day).

THINGS YOU CAN DO THIS WEEK

Load up on cruciferous vegetables on your next grocery run. Grab some broccoli, cauliflower, Brussels sprouts. Maybe even get some vegetables you are not used to eating, like Swiss Chard, collards, or bok choy, and aim to consume some at every meal for one week.

If insulin sensitivity is a concern, aim to go for a brisk walk after dinner tonight. A post-meal walk will help with the process of digestion, and because your bigger muscles (like your legs) are working, a lot of the carbohydrates from that meal will be deposited in these bigger muscles. If you consider yourself fit, try wearing a weighted vest for the walk. I have a fifteen-pound vest, and does it ever make a difference!

Get a full panel of blood, urine, and salivary testing done to establish where you are right now. This will help you assess objective changes in your hormones as you progress through perimenopause and menopause.

CHAPTER 6

THE BETTY EVENING: SLEEP AND SEX

The number one rule as a Betty is to protect your right to get a good night's rest. Sleep is the lynchpin for every other health desire you have, whether it is weight loss, better skin, more energy, improved ability to handle stress, or maintaining muscle mass. Sleep is the very first domino in being healthy. You cannot, and will not, be healthy, lose weight, or balance your hormones if you do not sleep well.

This is why I have organized the first step in your journey as cultivating an evening routine. Your evening rituals are a powerful tool to reduce stress from your day, honor the goddess within, and enjoy some private time so you can rest, relax, and win tomorrow. An evening routine not only honors the day you had, it prepares you for tomorrow by generating massive momentum, productivity, focus, creativity, and energy. Ending each day with gratitude, joy, and an intention to start the next day the way you want is how you reduce stress and engage in blissful rejuvenating sleep.

Setting up an evening routine is also a fundamental skill all women need in order to ramp up parasympathetic function (the branch of your nervous system that allows you to rest, an integral part of any evening). Good nightly routines lead to quality, deep, restorative sleep. Sleep is one of the primary ways you are going to heal.

Poor quality or quantity of sleep will affect every part of your humanity. If you do not sleep well, you cannot live well. You simply cannot be healthy without good sleep. If you do not sleep well, your body breaks down from a lack of good quality, restorative sleep.

Poor sleep has been shown to increase your appetite, often selectively more so for simple sugars and carbohydrates.[45] It impairs immune function by unnecessarily increasing pro-inflammatory pathways in the body.[46] It also increases blood pressure and impairs short- and long-term memory.[47] Lack of sleep is a stress response to our brains, and when we don't sleep, we go into survival mode.

The most common clinical presentations I see that coincide with poor sleep are obesity, hormonal imbalances, poor adaptation to stress, depression, anxiety, and physical misalignments such as back pain.[48]

Sleeping six hours or less per night will make you more insulin resistant, disrupt normal cortisol patterns, and decrease cognitive function.[49] This means your creativity, emotional regulation, and energy will be affected, not to mention you'll have a natural resistance to losing weight. Sleep deprivation facilitates exactly the opposite of what we are trying to achieve. Poor sleep affects everything. I must insist, Betty, that you get your rest.

WOMEN AND SLEEP

When we look at the stats, the picture of our collective poor sleep really comes to life. Fifty to seventy million Americans report sleep issues,[50] with insomnia reported as the most common sleep complaint. The ability to sleep is one of the most natural things on the planet and should be an effortless endeavor, both in initiation and maintenance.

There are myriad reasons falling and staying asleep can become difficult. Temperature regulation, hormones, menstrual cycle status, hot flashes, stress, obesity, timing of meals, alcohol, and snacking all affect sleep quality and function. It fares worse for those of us who travel across time zones for work. Constantly changing the timing of light and dark are deleterious to brain function, mental health, and performance.

With my female clients, I've observed a peculiar inverse relationship between sunset and anxiety. As the sun goes down, our anxiety levels begin to go up. We ruminate about the stresses we had today, the problems we are going to face tomorrow, all the things we didn't get done, and all the ways we failed. This leads to an inability to initiate sleep because our mind is racing, and over time, leads to an inability to maintain sleep because stress levels are high overnight.

In addition, sleep is a master regulator of women's hormones. Proper sleep leads to balanced testosterone levels, and even contributes to our sex drive![51] One study looked at sexual and genital response in women, and their data concluded that a one-hour increase in duration of sleep corresponded with a 13–15 percent increase in their interest in sex![52] As I have already alluded to in earlier chapters, I am a big fan of lots of orgasms for female health, and great sleep is how it starts, ladies!

Like our eating habits, our sleep requirements and quality will also change throughout our menstrual cycle. In your bleed week, you may find that as estrogen begins to rise, the quality of your sleep improves towards the end of that week. More sleep is especially important in the first half of our cycle, in the follicular phase. If we are sleep deprived in the follicular phase, it has been shown that we make greater errors in accuracy and memory, and we are less alert.[53]

Given that most women tend to have the most difficulty managing sleep in the second half of their cycle, needing more sleep in the first half of our menstrual cycle can seem surprising because we typically experience more sleep disturbances in our sleep cycles in the luteal phase. We experience more awakenings after sleep onset, a decrease in REM sleep, a decrease in total sleep time, and a decrease in sleep efficiency.[54]

Simply put, sleep *quality* is worse for us in the second half of our cycle.

Interestingly, though, studies consistently show that women in the luteal phase (despite our subjective, crappy sleep) have better accuracy and quicker reaction times than women in the follicular phase. At times, they even performed better than men, although you would expect that because of sleep disturbances, they would perform worse. Perhaps it is because progesterone, which is dominant in the luteal phase, increases the ability to maintain wakefulness and alertness.

Truthfully, you should be getting gorgeous, restorative sleep all the time, Betty. But if you are concerned about mental acuity and performance, pay particular attention to sleep in your follicular phase.

THE SLEEP-STARVED BRAIN EATS ITSELF

Many women I work with often acknowledge they should be getting more sleep, but work, family, travel, or all of the above interferes with their best intentions.

Now, here is where I need to, with loving and firm direction, *call you out on your excuses.* Your sleep *must* come first. It doesn't matter how clean your diet is, or how rock solid your exercise and training are. Sleep is the first domino for us Bettys. You simply cannot green smoothie and exercise your way out of bad sleep.

We discussed in Chapter 2 how chronic stress and inflammation preclude metabolic derangement, weight gain, and hormonal dysregulation. Poor sleep is a major contributor to chronic, low-grade inflammation and premature brain degeneration. You need to take sleep seriously.

The following paragraphs outline what happens when you do not get appropriate rest. Most shocking of all, you'll see, is the impact it has on brain structure and function. Poor sleep destroys your brain from the inside out.

In a super interesting study, Italian researchers looked at the effects of sleep deprivation on the brain.[55] They observed normal astrocyte activity in well-rested mice, with activity around 6 percent. *Astrocytes* are a part of the immune system in the brain and are responsible for clearing out toxic waste and debris. I think of astrocytes as the pool boys and landscape artists in the brain, pruning off old, unnecessary, unused synapses, and cleaning out brain gunk like plaques and cellular debris.

Normally, we want astrocytes to be active but not too active.

When they are overactive, they begin to prune healthy nerves, with a net result of reducing total volume in the brain. In chronically sleep-deprived mice, the activity of the astrocytes more than doubled. Chronic sleep deprivation in this study was defined as five days. Only five measly days! Does this sound familiar?

This study demonstrates how sleep deprivation can cause your brain to reduce its volume over time, meaning your brain gets smaller. When you are chronically sleep-deprived, those landscape artists in your brain become overactivated and over-zealous and will literally gnaw off and prune healthy synapses. The consequences of pulling all-nighters for exams or deadlines or having a bad week of sleep due to a sick child are greater than we thought.

ONE BAD NIGHT SLEEP = IMPAIRED MEMORY AND LEARNING

To make matters worse, just *one* bad night's sleep will not only affect the landscapers in the brain, but the function of an area of the brain called the *hippocampus*. The hippocampus is involved in consolidating learning, memories, and storing new memories. Sleep deprivation robs you of the ability to acquire new knowledge and shuts down your ability to retrieve information you already know.

Fat burning, fat loss, muscle gains, and learning take place when we have restful, uninterrupted sleep. Getting as little as six hours of sleep will cause declines in cognitive function, speed, and reaction time.

One study showed participants who had six hours of sleep per night performed as poorly as those who had had two nights of total sleep deprivation.[56] Perhaps the most shocking thing that emerged from this study was that the participants were largely unaware of the decline in their ability to perform cognitive tasks. In other words, they had significantly poorer function, *and were completely unaware of it.* They thought they performed just fine. Suffice it to say that, while you might think you can get by on six hours of sleep, the reality is, you cannot. Most people do not know how badly they are sleeping or the impact it had on their brain until they start sleeping better.

PLAQUES AND BRAIN CRUD

The final point I want to make around the deleterious effects of poor sleep come from the impact sleep deprivation has on your brain's ability to remove the build-up of cellular debris and plaquing every night. This is important because one of the things washed away nightly are *β-amyloid plaques*, the core proteins associated with Alzheimer's disease.

In our brain and throughout our nervous system, we have a sewage system called the *glymphatic system,* which is similar to the lymphatic system in the body. This system is designed to clean up and get rid of toxins that accumulate in the brain from everyday activity.[57] It essentially gives your brain a bath every night to remove the muck it accumulates from everyday life.

Imagine you have a curious toddler who loves to learn about her environment. She comes in from playing outside and is covered from head to toe in various debris. She has dirt lodged under her fingernails, mud on her knees, and every little nook and cranny of her body has something crudded on it. If you were to just take a showerhead and give her a quick wash down, you might clean some of the bigger areas, but you wouldn't get underneath the fingernails or in the nooks and crannies that need a good soak. The same is true for your brain. The longer you sleep, the longer you allow your glymphatic system to get into the crevices of the brain to remove the crud and gunk that build up every day.

When we sleep, our microglial cells (the pool boys and land-scapers we talked about earlier) shrink up to 200 percent in size to make room for cerebrospinal fluid to fill the brain, and wash out the "metabolic debris" of wakefulness.[58] We clear out plaques, tangles, and bits of debris and muck that are byprod-ucts of everyday living. If you cut your sleep short, you are effectively cutting short this necessary brain soak and will accu-mulate plaquing and debris faster than you can get rid of it. This, of course, has the cumulative effect over time of not only affecting brain health but accelerating brain aging.

SLEEP HABITS AND CIRCADIAN RHYTHMS

Another thing to note when thinking about restful sleep is that we are creatures of habit, and we maintain those habits via a daily clock called a *circadian rhythm*. Circadian rhythms are the cadence between the various internal "clocks" we have in our body and how they sync up to the master clock in our brain. This helps our master clock regulate our natural sleeping and waking cycles.

In general, we want to fall asleep and wake up at approximately the same time every day, just as you hear the familiar grumbling in your stomach at the same time every day signaling you to eat. Both of these are examples of our circadian biology at work.

The master "clock," the headmistress in our brain, is called the

Suprachiasmatic Nucleus (or SCN for short).[59] It is highly sensitive to light and directs and coordinates our wake and sleep cycles by evaluating how much light is coming through the retina. It also coordinates with other peripheral body-clocks using neural or hormonal signals, core body temperature, or eating and fasting cues.

You may already be familiar with blue-blocking glasses to reduce the amount of blue light our SCN detects. Hopefully, you are also beginning to see why late-night computer or device use, snacking, and large dinners throw off our internal clocks.

Let's walk through a common evening scenario for a working mom, keeping our internal clocks in mind.

SLEEPAGEDDON: A MODERN TALE OF EXHAUSTION

Outside, the sky begins to darken. This is a signal to our brain that it is time to start winding down. However, as is so common in our modern world, we remain on our phones, computers, and TVs well into the evening. For many of us, dinnertime is often the highest caloric intake of the day.

After dinner, maybe we watch TV, a Netflix special, or browse social media on our devices, continuing to increase the amount of light reaching our central clock in the brain. This exposure stops the natural release of melatonin,[60] our hormone of darkness. Another way to say this is by being on our devices, we are robbing our body's ability to initiate sleep.

Another scenario might be that we skip the screens, instead pouring ourselves a glass of wine or indulging in a late-night snack. Eating late at night has the same effect as being on screens. It creates circadian dissonance between the brain (which sees it's dark outside) and the body (which is now full of food to burn).[61]

When you eat late at night, the peripheral clocks in your liver, gut, and fat cells wake up—*Hey! There's new energy here! Time to rev things up and put this to good use!*—while your brain is like: *Whoa, but wait a minute…it's dark outside; isn't it time for bed?*

To address this modern problem, one of the best ways to reset and sync your clocks is to stop eating after seven o'clock in the evening. This allows the stomach several hours to empty (which is to say, while you are still upright and use gravity to aid in digestion) and sync up messages between your brain and body to wind down. Or, as a more general rule of thumb, stop eating three to four hours before bedtime to allow your stomach to empty itself completely before your nightly fast, and to help reduce your core body temperature.

In our household, all electronics (laptop, phone, TV) are closed at least two hours before bedtime, but we often have a "no device" rule from dinner onward. I also dim the lights so that the inside of the house mimics the lighting that is outside. Even in the dead of winter, when it gets dark by five o'clock in the evening, my family will sit down together and have dinner with the warm glow of candlelight.

I always tell my sons that the light inside the house should look like the light outside. When it is daytime, curtains are fully open, and lighting is on. In the evening, we match the light settings in the various rooms we are occupying to match what is happening outdoors. By mimicking the lighting of mother nature in your home, coupled with shutting down your devices an hour before bedtime, you now have a reasonable chance of initiating and engaging in the normal physiological process of sleep and healing your circadian biology.

While many people solely attribute melatonin as the sleep hormone, it is simply the forewoman who *initiates* sleep. Melatonin is often called the hormone of darkness, not because of any affiliation with Darth Vader (although that would be *awesome*), but rather because it is only secreted in the *absence* of light. This is why removing the stimulus of blue lights from our environment is so important, as being exposed to blue lights from our devices inhibits the release of melatonin. Melatonin has little influence on the *generation* of sleep, but the presence of melatonin coordinates different regions of the brain to initiate sleep.

Once sleep has begun, melatonin slowly decreases over the course of the night and into the morning. With light streaming into your bedroom window, this signals the brain to shut off melatonin production completely.

THE HORMONE OF GROGGINESS: ADENOSINE

For every minute you are awake, even as you read this book, adenosine is building up and accumulating in your brain. The longer you are awake, the more adenosine will accumulate. Once adenosine reaches a certain threshold, you will begin to feel groggy, and your desire for sleep will increase, something referred to as *sleep pressure*.

There is a way to get around this grogginess, of course, and I bet you've probably used this drug today or recently to help you wake up, be more alert, study, or reach a deadline. This drug, as you may have guessed, is caffeine.

Caffeine competes with adenosine on adenosine receptor sites to block adenosine's function.[62] Now, of course, caffeine, or as one of my patients lovingly called it, *hot brown water*, is one of the most abused psychoactive substances on the planet. You don't need to walk or drive very far to see a coffee shop ready to serve up this collective addiction.

Caffeine has a half-life of approximately six hours.[63] This means that it takes about six hours for your body to degrade this chemical in your body by half. Which, by extension, means it takes a *full twelve hours* to completely get rid of it. So, the cup of coffee you had at eleven o'clock in the morning can still be effectively blocking your adenosine receptors way into the evening, as late as eleven o'clock, the time when you want your sleep pressure and adenosine concentration to be at its peak.

Now, I love my morning hot brown water, the ritual around making it, the smell, and that first sip, but I also have genetics that afford me to metabolize caffeine quickly. So, instead of a half-life of six hours, my constitution allows my half-life clearance to be closer to four hours. Regardless of your genetic constitution, my best advice here is to have one cup of coffee in the morning, and that's it. Nix the afternoon coffee run at work. In Chapter 12, we'll explore other ways to level up your energy if you are feeling sluggish in the afternoon—ways that will not compromise the quality of your sleep later.

I've been tweaking my own nightly routine for a few years, and the best version so far is below. It has morphed considerably over time as my children have gotten older. My evening routine used to be me falling asleep as I nursed my child in a rocking chair. It has morphed to what you see below, given the current ages of my kidlets are ten and eight.

I expect this routine to continue to change with time as the needs of my children change. For most women, having an extended evening routine is nearly impossible. We are usually preparing dinner, helping kids complete homework, and preparing lunches for school the next day. I mention this *juuuust* in case you were tempted to blame yourself (as women tend to do) for not being able to journal endlessly in your bedroom in the evening. Anyone who has the liberty of doing so, I applaud this luxury, but it also means that someone else is tending to the children! With that in mind, use the following examples as a springboard for exploring what works for you.

THE BETTY EVENING ROUTINE
BUILD YOUR GREY MATTER

As with all rules, there is always at least one juicy exception. I have been lamenting about the mechanics of sleep, and the detriment of blue light exposure to our circadian biology for good reason. However, playing videos games has been shown to grow areas of the brain involved in memory and learning. There are many video games to choose from, but spatial puzzle solving games like Tetris and even Super Mario 64 have been shown to increase the volume of nerves in your hippocampus.[64]

In other words, adding a puzzle game to your routine helps support your brain's adaptability and flexibility—two crucial tools shown to help combat prominent neurodegenerative diseases like Alzheimer's, multiple sclerosis, and dementia.

Playing Tetris has been shown to increase the volume of our grey matter (the place where our nerve cells start). There's even a name for it: The Tetris Effect. An interesting study looked at MRI brain scans for two categories of adolescent girls: those who played Tetris for thirty minutes a day, and those who did not.[65] After three months, the participants who played Tetris had thicker grey matter than they did when the experiment began. Playing Tetris has also been shown to improve both long-term and working memory, spatial awareness, and depth perception. It also helps amplify your problem-solving abilities by regularly encouraging you to look at situations from various perspectives.

So, we work this video game into your evening routine by playing the game well in advance of your bedtime and putting on some stylish blue-light blocking glasses.

CREATE AN ELECTRONIC-FREE BEDROOM

We are electromagnetic beings. Our brain sends electrical impulses down through the spinal cord, to our peripheral nerves, to every inch of our body. Our brain also receives information about the body from our sensory nerves. These detect everything from temperature and pressure to vibration, proprioception, and more. Our central and peripheral nervous systems are electric. Our hearts have an even greater electromagnetic field than our brain, and your heart beats due to an electric pulse from the pacemaker buried within its structure.

Bathing your cells in the electromagnetic radiation from televisions, phones, and other devices will affect your quality of sleep, particularly your HRV, or *heart rate variability*. Heart rate variability is the variability in timing between each heartbeat. Although counterintuitive, you want irregularity in your heart rate because it signals a balance in both the sympathetic and parasympathetic branches of your nervous system.

One of the easiest ways to get rid of excess electromagnetic radiation is to ban all devices (including the TV on the wall) from your room. Charge your phones in the kitchen and get rid of any Bluetooth speakers in your room. In fact, I would make it a habit to turn off Bluetooth whenever you are not using it and shut down your home's Wi-Fi signal at night.

RAISE EVENING OXYGEN LEVELS

So, what are you supposed to do if you cannot scroll on your phone or binge Netflix in the evening?

Consider for a moment that in a healthy individual, oxygen saturation rates should be 98 to 100 percent during the day, and as evening approaches, oxygen saturation can begin to fall by 4 to 5 percent.[66]

This has direct implications for our heart function. If we have less oxygen saturation, we can expect other vital markers, like heart rate, to be impacted over time. When your cells don't get adequate oxygen, your heart has to work harder to pick up the slack. The adaptive response to less oxygen in the body is an elevated heart rate.

Tachycardia, or an elevated heart rate, is one of the earliest signs of cardiovascular stress, and eventually impacts blood pressure.[67] If your heart rate is chronically elevated because of poor oxygenation, the blood vessels and their resistance to stretch will be negatively impacted over time, as well.

Remember, as a woman, cardiovascular disease is still our number one killer. Taking good care of your heart, especially in the hours before you go to sleep, is so important! So, one of the easiest ways to keep your heart healthy (and not overworked) is to make sure you are well oxygenated in the evening.

One of the easiest ways to improve oxygen levels in the evening is to take a light, brisk walk or engage in some light stretching or breathwork. We've already talked about how this aids in digestion, and another perk will be to oxygenate your body in preparation for a restful night's sleep.

If you want to monitor your oxygen levels, an oximeter is an easy purchase from Amazon or any online retailer. If the weather precludes you from walking outside, invest in a walking treadmill. I have one that I use at my desk, and in fact, I am walking at 1.5 mph as I type this. If you are tracking your steps with a pedometer, aim for at least four thousand steps after dinner, or the equivalent of a thirty-minute walk. This will help your posture, strengthen your heart and big muscles like your legs, and improve dilation of your arteries and their ability to get vital blood to your cells![68]

As I mentioned in Chapter 2, carving out time for focused breath work in the evening can help with lowering stress and allows you to prepare for a restful slumber.[69] To do this, sit in a comfortable, crossed-legged position with your back supported and start with circle breaths. With your mouth open, take in a large quantity of air for one breath, allowing your belly to expand. Without pausing at the top, begin exhaling, making a loud "ah" or sighing noise. I will often listen to a music playlist (with my phone on airplane mode) and practice this breathing anywhere from three to forty-five minutes while my kids are playing in the backyard. Be forewarned, though—this type of circle breathing is a trip! You may feel tingly all over, almost like you are high. This is an effective way to improve oxygen and should feel really great.

Another way to relax in the evening is by doing gentle stretches or yoga. One of my favorite ways to transition into the evening is to do a yoga class. I always find if I can get it in before dinnertime, it is the best. I tend to prefer the traditional sun salutation sequences found in Ashtanga and Hatha Yoga practices. For women who are chronically stressed, I also suggest Yin Yoga, where the asanas are held for longer periods of time. This helps connective tissue like our fascia and joints release tension.

You can also add plants to your bedroom like snake plants or aloe vera.[70] These plants typically absorb carbon dioxide overnight and release oxygen into the bedroom air, providing an oxygen-rich sleeping environment.

GRATITUDE JOURNALING

To relax for the evening, I also spend five minutes answering the following questions:

What were three amazing things that happened today?

What's one (or two) thing(s) I learned today?

Simply said, these exercises reduce the gnawing anxiety that is waiting to come out and steal your sleep. The neurophysiology behind these exercises is that they get you out of your limbic system and into your neocortex.[71] The limbic system is responsible for our emotions, among other things. The limbic system is hardwired for survival. As such, it's where our fearful thoughts reside. Often called our lizard brain, it is primarily concerned with survival.

When we are in our limbic system, we might find ourselves

using words like *always* and *never* ("My daughter *never* says thank you," or "My husband *always* leaves the housework to me"). The limbic system deals in absolutes, and there is never any nuance to it. When we are emotionally triggered or tired, our limbic system can take over if we are not conscious of it. When I'm beginning to sound nasally, whiny, and annoyed at everyone, I ask myself, "Hey Steph…do you think you are tired?"

Brain expert Dr. Daniel Amen calls these thoughts ANTs, or Automatic Negative Thoughts. As you may have guessed from the name, we can't control these thoughts. No number of ohms or chanting will get rid of them. You cannot stop your brain from thinking involuntarily, just like you cannot stop your heart from beating involuntarily. But we can change the thoughts we choose to focus on.

These journaling exercises are what I like to call "frontal lobe flex exercises" in disguise. They will selectively bias you out of your limbic system and into the higher centers of your brain that are involved in gratitude, happiness, and joy. This is why gratitude is so powerful. Actively looking for things that are great in your life will help you continue to notice more great things in your life. This is you taking the reins and directing your brain towards what to focus on.

By default, we tend to have a lot of negative thoughts, and they can turn very quickly into catastrophizing thoughts. In order to turn this around, we need to believe in a better thought. It doesn't have to be a magical, sparkly, perfect thought; it just needs to be better than the catastrophe.

If you screamed at your kids, lost it on a client, and forgot to feed the dog, journaling that you remained calm all day long is not going to resonate because you know it is not true, and therefore will not have the neurochemical cascade you are looking for. Your brain can be a hostile cross-examining lawyer and will pick apart everything you say. In the scenario above, you might say, I am grateful for the opportunity to look at why I was triggered with my kids today, to better understand my own trauma, and I learned that when I only sleep for six hours, I am short-tempered.

The key here is these journaling exercises are short, sweet, and to the point. You don't need to write a novella each evening. If you are having trouble thinking of things to be grateful for, get back to the basics. You are grateful to have woken up this morning, for your family, for your career, for your dog, for your nails, and for implementing everything Dr. Stephanie says in this book. OK, maybe that last one is mine, but hopefully you get the picture of this quick and efficient exercise.

REFRAME NEGATIVE EXPERIENCES

I always follow the exercise above with these two questions to ponder:

What's one thing you could have handled better today?

What is one word to describe how I want to show up tomorrow?

This is a practice of forgiveness, humility, and self-actualization. We all make mistakes, and we all regress to fear, anger, or behaviors that we are less than proud of. It is a complete waste of time beating yourself up about what happened. What is a great use of your time is reflecting upon why it did happen, and how you can improve for the next situation that presents itself. I am a firm believer that you are never given anything you cannot handle. It may mean the acquisition of new skills, an up-leveling in your thought, and for you to sit with some uncomfortable feelings, but if you focus on improvement, improvement is what you will gain. Being honest with yourself, with a loving, gentle hand, is how you can step into who you already are and be more of yourself.

Channeling a word that embodies your highest self is something I borrowed from Danielle Laporte, a member of Oprah's Super-Soul 100. Danielle has created books, planners, and courses on how to channel what she calls "core desired feeling." So many of us have "to do" lists, but how do we want to feel when we do them? What words come to mind? Strong? Calm? Peaceful? Luminous? Graceful? Sexy? Alive? Tender? The world of words is your oyster here. Consult a thesaurus for some inspiration and think of what embodying that word means for *you*.

If you had a challenging encounter with a co-worker, family member, or friend today and didn't express yourself or behave the way you wish you had, mentally re-enact the scenario in the way *the best version of yourself would have handled it*. A gentle reminder for my feisty Bettys, this is not an opportunity to use your best one-liner. This exercise is designed to help prime you to act in accordance with the best version of yourself.

Parenting expert Jennifer Kolari, author of *Connected Parenting*, once said to me if it feels good to say something in the moment, it is probably the wrong thing to say. You know the one. The well-timed insult, the thing you've been rehearsing to say to your partner, the argument you've been having in your head all day with that one person. If you have the perfect one-liner in your head, you've already lost. For me, this is often something I reflect upon in the context of my role as a parent. I think about how I could have better showed up for my kids, where I could have improved my behavior, and how I could have showed them more compassion.

If I didn't show up the way I wanted, I will replay the scenario as if I *did* act the way I wanted to. This can also be done in the context of your romantic relationship as well. When you reframe a negative experience by visualizing yourself acting as your highest self, the brain begins to create neural pathways that will be available to you when a similar scenario puts you to the test. And it will. This reflection and visualization will prime you to get it right next time.

CHUCK YOUR PILLOW

Another way to induce blissful rejuvenating sleep, not to mention promote proper spinal alignment, is by reducing pillow use. When you are sleeping, you are designed to move into a variety of positions all night long. This includes on your back, on your side, and, yes, even on your stomach.

Let's engage a little experiment to demonstrate. Wherever you are now, roll your shoulders forward, let your chin fall forward, and round your upper back. Take a deep breath in and notice how it feels. Now, roll your shoulders back and down, bring your chin back up and slightly tip it up, and straighten your upper back. Take another deep breath in.

Which of these two scenarios felt easier?

I'm guessing the second one was easiest. This is because when you are in extension, you allow for more room for expansion in your thoracic cavity. The ribs roll and open, the diaphragm is not being crushed, so it can depress, and your throat's capacity to take in oxygen is amplified.

If you sleep with a pillow under your neck while sleeping on your back, you are putting your neck into flexion, and constricting airway flow. If you have ever taken a cardiorespiratory resuscitation (CPR) course, one of the first interventions is to open the airway, and this is done by extending the neck to tilt the head up.

The narrative we often hear is that we need to keep our spine "aligned" with a good pillow. I beg to differ. A working knowledge of spinal mechanics and its interplay with aging reveals why the use of a pillow may be a contributing factor to a hypoxic brain environment. The two motions in the neck we lose as we age are extension and rotation. Which means sleeping in a position that will naturally encourage extension, rotation, or both simultaneously will naturally benefit the neck and breathing. And extension and rotation of the neck promote the natural and necessary curve of the neck, referred to as *lordosis*. Lordosis in the neck and the low back is essentially a backward "C" curve that is needed for proper movement, symmetry, joint loading, and to protect the spinal cord that is housed inside the spine.

Sleeping on your back with a pillow induces flexion into the spine, but you already have alllllllll the flexion you need. You're in flexion all day every day while you are awake.

For the most part, we spend our days in a flexed, hunched over position. Think about it. You sit in your car or on the subway on your way to work. You then sit at your desk, working steadily at your computer for twelve to sixteen hours. You might go to a restaurant at lunch where you sit, and then return to sit at your desk. Then, we drive or sit on our way back home. We sit for dinner. We sit on the couch and watch TV. Over the course of time, spending many hours in this position will cause your spine to begin to deform into a flexed, or hyperkyphotic state.

The term I am describing is known as *creep*. And, no, not the weird guy from your office. Physiological creep is a phenomenon where your muscles, ligaments, and joints will start assuming the flexed position, *even when you are not in that position.*[72]

We all know someone whose posture is so poor that it seems like their head walks into the room before they do. I think of some of the elder patients I have cared for over the years. With time, their heads are so far forward, they seem permanently stuck there. And while this anterior head carriage used to be confined only to the elderly, I have had cases of eight- and nine-year-old kids in my practice with flattened spines from excessive screen time. Sleeping supine (on your back) with a pillow simply mimics and reinforces the flexion from the day. Computers are not going anywhere, so we must learn to undo the damage we incur during the day at night.

What we know about postural distortion is that it is linked to higher mortality rates.[73] So first things first…ditch the pillows if you like sleeping on your back. This will naturally induce a mild extension in the neck (which, structurally, you need for normal mechanical function), and more importantly will not create more flexion in your day.

STOMACH SLEEPING

I reject the idea that we should sleep in one position all night long, or that there are "good" sleep positions and "bad" sleep positions. This includes stomach sleeping. Stomach sleeping can and should be celebrated as an easy and natural way to rehab your neck overnight!

If you stop to think about what happens when you sleep on your stomach, your head is in slight extension, and it is rotated to one side. You are effectively introducing the very movements you don't get enough of during the day. The deep and superficial flexion muscles of the neck are getting lengthened, and the muscles in the back of the neck are being shortened. This is precisely what we want to see when looking at balance and symmetry of these opposing muscle groups.

If you can slowly and methodically train yourself to get comfortable sleeping on your stomach, then you have unlocked the secret bonus level of neck health, and potentially avoid brain fog by inducing a better night's sleep through improving oxygen uptake. Stomach sleeping encourages diaphragmatic breathing, which can reduce hypoxia.[74] It also has the bonus of toning and strengthening your diaphragm because it needs to work against your own natural body to depress. The diaphragm is not only important in respiration but in spinal stability and in the strength of your core muscles. As we sleep on our stomachs, we strengthen part of our core.

If sleeping on your stomach is difficult for you, start slowly. Spend a minute or two on your belly with your head turned to one side, and then the equivalent with your head to the other. You will naturally move into all sorts of positions overnight, and that is totally normal. Undoing the flexor dominance in your neck can take time, and giving your body the time to adapt is important. If it is available to you, you can also work this in with a chiropractor or bodyworker you trust who is well aware of the consequences of poor spinal curves and mechanics. Being adjusted helps improve the mobility, flexibility, and symmetry of your muscles and the bones of the spine.

OH, THE PLACES YOU WILL GO WITH THE BIG "O"

I'll just get straight to the point here. Ladies, you need to be climaxing as often as you can. Whether it is with your partner, or a toy you call your partner, get after those orgasms! For women, this is a crucial piece of our health puzzle that we often miss, because we are too busy, forget, or feel an incredible amount of shame around orgasms.

If we think about female anatomy, one of our unique features is that there is no other function for the clitoris other than pleasure. Clocking in with a whopping eight thousand nerve endings, double that of the penis, it has absolutely no reproductive function. Yet another reason to love being a woman, right?

The male equivalent would be the penis, which has many roles, including reproduction, pleasure, and urination. In a woman, these functions are divided into separate anatomical areas. You might (accurately) deduce then, that as a woman, pleasure is your birthright, and in your inherent design.[75]

Depending on the learned patterns from your family or culture of origin, this might fly squarely in the face of your deeply held beliefs. And the reality is most cultures view woman as the weaker and more insignificant of the two sexes. A common conservative structure of a male-female dyad might be the woman is tasked with the child-rearing, housework, and cooking.

Now let me be clear—this is not a commentary about what is 'right' or 'wrong,' but my experience tells me that in these pursuits, a woman often forgets about her own needs. She gets lost in the homework, the soccer schedule, the meal prep, and the demands at work. She forgets the things that bring her pleasure. This not only pertains to her sexual pleasure, but the pleasure that comes from taking care of herself. Viewing herself as someone worth worshipping, worth getting to know, and worth taking care of is a journey most women do not awaken to. You have picked up this book for a reason, and my guess would be that in part, it is because somewhere inside there is a voice that says you are worth getting to know in every way.

Let me build the case for why you need to get to know your clitoris and why you need boatloads of orgasms.

Aside from being a great cardiovascular workout, orgasms improve circulation to the pelvic cavity and reduce chronic stress and sympathetic dominance by restoring balance to the autonomic nervous system. In order to climax, you must activate both the sympathetic and parasympathetic nervous systems.

This better blood flow and neurological balance will promote healthy estrogen metabolism. Remember Estrogen's Gold Rule: use it and then lose it! You want to use it, and then get rid of it efficiently. This is especially important if you are in peri-menopause, where there is an initial tendency to run estrogen dominant (see Chapter 4 for a review on estrogen dominance).

The knock-on effect of improving estrogen metabolism is it will also help to regulate your menstrual cycle. Studies have shown that women who have sex once per week are more likely to have normal menstrual cycles, including less cramping, bloating, and symptoms of PMS than those who are celibate or have infrequent sex.[76]

Orgasms flush out cortisol, one of our stress hormones, and induce a deep sense of relaxation and bliss by boosting endorphin levels, oxytocin, and increasing pain tolerance. And if that wasn't enough, orgasms make you look younger. Oh, yes, Betty. The Big O has anti-aging properties.[77]

Sounds like it's worth getting to know yourself a little better, right? I cannot emphasize this enough: you need an orgasm on the regular, Betty. Let's call it twice weekly (at a minimum) to start. Or maybe a fun experiment might be a seven-day orgasm challenge. You can see how it will change your mood, your energy, and even your face! Take a picture of your face before you start your seven-day challenge, and then one at the very end. What changes do you notice?

Remember pleasure is your birthright, and it is yours to enjoy. No matter what your sexual orientation, religious or spiritual beliefs, the science doesn't lie. There is a reason you have a clitoris—eight thousand reasons, in fact—one for each nerve ending.

TO VIBRATE OR NOT TO VIBRATE?

As you can see, there are a myriad of ways regular orgasms can help your hormones, your weight loss efforts, the way your body feels, and your brain. But there is a difference between an orgasm from a vibrator, and one from your hands.

How we climax is also just as important as *how often* we do.

Using toys are great—they add variety, and are, *ahem*, an efficient way to get the job done. You can usually climax quite quickly, which can be convenient if you are in between meetings, tired at the end of a long day, or the threat of kids bursting into your bedroom does not afford a lot of time for self-exploration.

But if that becomes the *only* way you are experiencing orgasms, you are missing out on some of the massive health benefits and the opportunity to get to know yourself and what you like. You will also struggle to show your partner what you like and don't like.

There are four distinct phases to an orgasm: excitement, plateau, orgasm, and resolution. And the way we orgasm is different depending on how we are stimulated.

Excitement

This is when your heart rate and blood pressure start climbing, and you may notice a reddening of the skin around your chest and neck. Nitric oxide begins to be released, causing the tension in our muscles to relax, and dramatically increases the blood supply to the vagina and cervix. The extra blood flow then triggers vaginal lubrication, and general muscle tension begins to build up.

Plateau

This is the phase of most importance, and the distinguishing factor between an orgasm achieved manually or mechanically. In this phase, there is increased activity in pleasure centers in the brain, like the amygdala and the hippocampus. Anxiety centers in the brain shut down, and we are able to experience more dopamine and adrenaline. This is where we experience increased pain and stress tolerance (which is really great if you suffer from a lot of cramping and tenderness around the onset of your period). The muscle tension from the excitement phase is now being transformed into contractions and muscle spasms in body parts like your hands, feet, and face.

Orgasm

The peak! Here, your heart rate, breathing rate, and blood pressure are all at their peak. There is a marked increase in the production and release of oxytocin. This causes the uterus to contract, working to help semen get drawn up through the cervix. The muscles of the pelvic floor are now contracting somewhere between five to twelve times per second.

Resolution

The heart rate, muscular tension, and respiratory rate all begin to return to normal. Oxytocin rushing in creates that post-orgasmic glow, and melatonin is released, which is why we often feel sleepy afterwards.

You can see why if a mechanical toy is the *only* source of your orgasms, you will consistently bypass the *plateau* phase of your orgasm. This bypasses the hormone balancing effects of several hormones like testosterones, estrogens, and many others. If you are already dealing with a hormonal imbalance discussed in Chapter 3, a manual climax can (and should) be one of the regular ways you experience orgasms.

If it has been a hot minute since you have experienced a manual orgasm, here are a few suggestions to get started:

- Choose a time, say once a week, where you can allow extra time for play.
- Environment matters! Treat your bedroom like it is hosting the goddess it is. Pick the clothes off the floor, dim the lights, and moisturize your body with coconut oil.
- Have some essential oils on hand, such as clary sage, lavender, sandalwood, rose, or ylang ylang to diffuse into the air. All are reported to have female-arousal properties.
- Draw a warm bath and drop some essential oils into the bathwater.
- Take a direct sniff of rose essential oil at the end of the day, in the quiet of your bedroom.
- Read erotica.
- Use a natural lubricant like coconut oil and spend time learning about yourself and getting to know what you like.

THINGS YOU CAN DO THIS WEEK

Commit to eight hours of sleep per night, starting tonight! You can also reduce technology use in the hours leading up to bed, dim the lights in the house to match the external environment, and wear blue-blocking glasses that will promote a healthy, rejuvenating sleep.

Download Tetris on your phone and start playing daily, ideally while it is still light outside.

Keep a gratitude journal and start looking for the smallest things you can be appreciative of, even if it is as simple as, "I woke up this morning."

When negative things happen (they always will!), reframe them as an opportunity to learn from them rather than beat yourself up. Every missed win is a message to go within to understand your triggers and patterns.

Orgasm twice weekly at a minimum. And if you feel up to it, take the Seven-Day Orgasm Challenge!

CHAPTER 7

MASTERPIECE LIVES START WITH MASTERPIECE MORNINGS: COLD TATAS AND WATER WITH BENEFITS

There is something about your favorite dress or pair of jeans that makes you feel like a million bucks. The way it hugs your curves and accentuates your shape to instantly give you confidence, grace, and ease with the way you move, and even the way you stand. This is but a mere piece of clothing, yet it feels fabulous on your body and knows how to move with you. Surprisingly, it also has confidence-boosting effects on your mind. Having a morning routine is like putting on your favorite pair of jeans every day. It allows you to admire all that is great about you, calms your anxiety about any perceived flaws, and gives you the confidence to step into your day powerfully.

A morning routine is a must for any Betty who wants to feel good in her body and radiate from within. And I am the first to admit I used to turn my nose up at morning routines, thinking these were pastimes of the worried well, or for women who had too much time on their hands. After all, my stress is what drives me, makes me produce, and achieve all that I have, right?

It took me years (OK, fine, decades) to begin to unhitch my need (OK, fine, addiction) to stress and my perception around productivity. I always thought my stress was what made me successful. What would happen to me if I gave up my habit of being stressed out? Would I relax and become a sloth? Or worse, would I become…unproductive?! After speaking to thousands of women about this, I know these musings are not mine alone.

Countless women have become addicted to being stressed out, even though we understand what stress does to us. It makes your brain smaller and sets you up for weight gain, inflammation, and hormonal derangement.[78] This is why we need to set ourselves up to start our days from a place of peace.

Developing sacred rituals and rhythms will calm you down, help decrease your stress response (which we discussed in Chapter 2), and create resilience. It will teach you to be present, sharpen your brain, and, most of all, propel you toward the goals you have set for yourself in your life. And if that goal is weight loss, then you absolutely must develop a morning routine you love, and one you can easily do most days.

Practicing morning rituals and rhythms regularly will also have several knock-on effects as well. Your calmer behavior will be noticed and modeled by your children. They will see your interest in self-development and growth, and this will become a new "normal" for them, leading them to internalize these behaviors. It will have knock-on effects on your relationship with your partner and allow for new levels of connection and growth as a couple. You will be calmer, and dare I be bold enough to say you will be happier and enjoy your body.

This morning ritual is a time that will honor you, your body, and your mind. Let's be honest, you give of yourself to so many people. In order to do that effectively, you need to love up on yourself, too. Remember the instruction from the safety demonstration on an airplane that says to put on your own oxygen mask before assisting others. Most women completely forget about their own needs; instead placing all other commitments ahead of their own.

The idea of self-care can be confusing. It has somehow morphed into this idea of manicures and bubble baths. While these are definitely part of self-care, they are more of a luxurious add-on to the fundamentals we will discuss here.

The key to success with a morning routine is ease and consistency. Ease is designed around something you can do every day and can easily adapt to the day or week you are having. Consistency comes after you've practiced (and failed) a lot. You don't get a shredded body by doing one bicep curl. You don't get healthy by eating one salad. You practice, you repeat, and you do things routinely until they are second nature. And your healthy practices benefit you over the long term when done consistently. Practice makes progress.

There is no one perfect morning routine. And if we are being perfectly honest here, most morning routines are blatantly sexist. I cannot tell you how many morning routines I have read about and have not been able to implement because I have young children, only to realize all the routines were created by men. You know, these two-hour rituals wherein you wake up at an ungodly hour to make special tea, followed by endless journaling, working out for an hour, and then reading fifty pages in a book before ever checking an email. Uh...have you ever heard a woman touting this? I have yet to come across a woman with such a routine, yet there are books dedicated to waking up earlier than early and creating a stagnant, stringent morning routine *no matter what.*

Except these books omit this one, itty bitty, tiny little detail: most of these rituals are practiced and preached by men. If said men have a family with children, it is their partner who is taking care of the kids and running the house while he can luxuriate in his morning routine. And if he is able to, good for him. This just isn't a possibility for many women who are single moms, or even those in a partnership because the bulk of the caregiving still falls on the woman.

My routines have evolved as my children have gotten older. It used to be a child woke me up, and then I tended to them until they went down for their nap. Then and only then did I try to sneak in something for myself. In those early days of motherhood, if I was waking myself up at five o'clock in the morning to journal, my head would have exploded. So, go easy on yourself, and figure out where you are right now, and what works for you.

I want to redefine what it means to have a morning routine, because some days my morning routine involves my kids piling into my bed to cuddle, and other times I bring them downstairs with me to squeeze in a forty-five-minute workout. And in the spirit of being totally honest with you, sometimes I miss my morning routine altogether. This is not about being perfect. This is about designing a morning routine and figuring out what works and what doesn't.

Think of your morning ritual practice as a way to start your day with some kind of win, however small. Sometimes, my win is putting my favorite oils on my face, and other times, it is my full workout plus a meditation session. It is all perfectly imperfect.

There are three basics I like to try and get in *at some point* in my morning routine. This can be all at once or staggered between breakfast, packing lunches, and school drop off. It can happen in increments, and I usually try to get them in at some point before noon, according to my schedule and energy that day.

These basics are rehydration, movement, and cold showers. I have chosen these because they have been shown time and again to help you look and feel younger, energize your cells, awaken your brain, lower inflammation, and develop cellular grit.[79] Every Betty needs these benefits in the morning when trying to manage the house, get the kids to school, and head out the door for work!

WATER WITH BENEFITS

Technically, we all fast for eight hours overnight while we sleep. Upon waking, the first thing on the list is to rehydrate your body. I strongly prefer water and the practice of rehydration in the mornings over food. I will provide more detail about this in Chapter 10 when we discuss fasting, but for now, know that water trumps food first thing in the morning.

I keep a pitcher of water by my nightstand and can usually drink a glass immediately upon waking. If time affords it, I will then proceed to drink 750 mL (about ¾ of a quart) of water. And I'll be honest, I have struggled with drinking water my whole life. I have resisted because there is no taste to water, and I find it boring. What I have learned is to pep it up and pretend like I'm in a spa. Making it seem like a treat is the only way I am going to get it done. I infuse the water with cucumber slices or limes, or even blueberries and mint leaves. I put it in an ornate pitcher on a beautiful tray on my nightstand. That way, I awaken to a little treat first thing upon waking.

And water is one of those basics that we all know we need to get better at, but we just don't.

I feel like you may not be fully convinced, so let me try and drive this point home. The more water you drink, the more your body will let go of the water you are carrying. The more water you consume, the plumper and fuller your face will look (say bye-bye fine lines and wrinkles!). When you are hydrated, this signals to the body to let go of extra water.[80]

Hunger and thirst often feel the same in the body.[81] In fact, in my online nutrition program, we talk about this extensively: if you feel you might be hungry, grab an 8- to 10-ounce glass of water and wait twenty minutes. If you are still hungry, then your signals were truly hunger. If the grumbling goes away, it was dehydration. More often than not, it is lack of water that drives what seems to be hunger. But always remember, hunger and thirst *feel* like the same thing. It is your job to figure out which one it is. Making sure you are getting enough water will help you whittle down consumption of empty calories, and help you stop searching the fridge for the tenth time looking for something to quell the grumbling in your stomach.

Commit to two liters (about two quarts) of water every single day.[82] Spread it out over the course of the day. Your body will be well hydrated and begin to let go of excess water. Be forewarned—you will pee a lot initially, but as you shed the excess water, your trips to the bathroom will return to normal. You can get creative and put mint, cucumber, blueberries, and limes in the water, whatever you love. Your plump skin, full lips, and lack of belly bloat with thank you for it.

MOVEMENT

Physical priming in the morning is simply choosing movement (any movement) and doing it. Push-ups, jumping jacks, squats, lunges, sit-ups, handstands, rebounders, a morning walk, some stretches, or dance to your favorite song…anything you want. The point is to just pick something and do it. Something. Anything. Just move!

You can choose twenty reps of any exercise, or ten minutes of dancing like nobody's watching. Put on some tunes and GO! This burst of exercise in the morning is perfect, as it helps to balance out curves in cortisol and drive up energy production.[83]

Movement is one of the fundamental basics I use to help women reclaim their energy. All you need is five minutes of full-body movement to get this process started. If you have time for a longer workout, that's great, too! This physical movement, even if it is short, creates massive momentum for your ability to think, ideate, and create. It is a powerful cognitive priming.[84]

Performing short bursts of activity is a quick win, and it wakes up your frontal lobe (the area where creativity, focus, and decision-making live) by lighting up the motor, premotor, and prefrontal cortex. This is a great hack to get you into a state of flow.

For most of us, our peak productivity is in the morning, a few hours after waking. Your brain is the most awake and has the most juice in the tank, which can be amplified with movement in the morning.[85] That way, you'll have more resilience to deal with whatever happens for the rest of the day, whether it be a work deadline or family emergency.

I have played with movements to figure out what suits my body best in the morning. Personally, I love a hard workout in the morning—either a weight workout or burst training. If you are short on time, put on one or two of your favorite songs, and just dance! Something is better than nothing. It doesn't have to be elaborate; you just have to move!

COLD TATAS

Brutal truth time here—I started off absolutely hating the idea of a cold shower. I thought, what could be worse than a freezing shower? Nothing. Nothing could be worse. My Mediterranean genes demand sun and heat, damnit! But I could not deny the data supporting cold showers: energy production, mitochondrial biogenesis, reduced brain fog, and anti-aging skin benefits.[86]

So, I begrudgingly started my experiment with myself as the only participant to see if this made a difference for me. I decided to start slowly and work my way up. A five-minute, ice-cold shower seemed like an eternity, so I decided to end my normal shower with thirty seconds of cold. And I'm going to be straight-up honest—I felt like a drowning cat with no escape.

But now, immediately after I get through one to two minutes of a cold shower, the effects are undeniable. I am brighter, more sparkly, shinier, and more awake. It works. So, I try to remember that the cold shower is akin to that first jump in the lake on summer holidays. Whenever I go to the beach, the water starts off *freezing*. And then you just get used to it after a while.

WHAT YOU CAN DO THIS WEEK

Treat yourself to a lemon-infused pitcher of water on your nightstand. Tomorrow, first thing, drink one cup. You can get creative and mix in cucumbers, lemons, limes, and even blueberries!

Think of how you can start your day off with movement every morning. It can be a full workout or a five-minute dance break.

Pinky promise yourself to try cold water for the last five seconds of your next shower.

CHAPTER 8

BECOMING A FAT BURNER IN TWENTY-EIGHT DAYS

At this point, my hope is you are creating sacred morning and evening rituals, your sleep is slowly improving, and you might even feel like you have a squeak more energy. Now, at this point in your healing, we'll tackle your metabolism. Specifically, we are going to turn you into a fat-burning machine, increase your energy, and help you feel full while doing it. You, Betty, are now ready for a dive into ketosis.

Metabolic flexibility is the ability to switch from being a sugar burner to a fat burner. Most of us stay in a sugar-burning mode and never truly open up our fat reserves for energy use. This next part of our journey will train your cellular machinery to easily use fat for energy production. The word 'ketogenic' refers to our bodies' production of ketone bodies, which are derived from fat and can be used instead of glucose to make energy in the cell, with fewer byproducts and waste. Ketone bodies can be a more efficient fuel source for the brain and can help reduce the production of free radicals when compared to using glucose as an energy precursor[87].

Unlike other ketogenic diets, this way of eating will help you lose weight without being hungry.[88] This approach is sustainable rather than designed for short-term gains like many other diets. And honestly, I have little interest in short-terms gains. What is the point of doing all this work if the results are only temporary?! I am interested in playing the long game with your health, so when you lose the weight, you can keep it off.

THE ESTIMA DIET (TWENTY-EIGHT DAYS OF KETOSIS)

The first part of regaining your metabolism is a twenty-eight-day, or four-week, female-focused, ketogenic diet. This length of time is the first step, no matter your age and menstrual status. This phase of the program is designed for fat loss. So, you can repeat this four-week cycle as often as you'd like to achieve your goal. Once it has been achieved, move into the cyclic ketogenic eating pattern outlined in Chapter 9.

Based on experience, most women typically need to prioritize fat loss through ketosis for ninety days, or about three cycles of The Estima Diet. At the end of each cycle, you will record your weight and measurements in the Weight Tracker, found in the appendix section of this book.

If you have never engaged in a ketogenic diet, or if you have and found you couldn't stick with it, I am excited for your results. So many women come to me either unsure how to implement it or have tried and fallen off the wagon. For the most part, it is because the keto diets they have tried in the past consist of bacon, butter, and burgers on eternal repeat. There were no green vegetables to be found, no resistant starches to quell their cravings and heal their microbiome, and loads of processed or saturated fats. This protocol is different. There will be no tubs of sour cream to devour, no bacon on bacon with a side of bacon. You will consume lots of leafy green vegetables, high-quality proteins, and lots of heart-healthy fats.

On a cellular level, eating a properly formulated, high-fat, low-carb diet will support enhanced mitochondrial function. This will amp up your ability to produce energy.[89] Because we are tapping into producing our own ketones, it will reduce oxidative damage from free radicals and help you lose excess fat.

The standard American diet (aptly abbreviated "SAD") is full of processed carbohydrates and trans fats, and both are often rolled into one product. Referred to as "bliss point" foods, these foods are highly addictive, nutrient-devoid toxic garbage. Even a prominent chip manufacturer boasts their addictive nature in slogans like, "Betcha can't eat just one!" They know their food is addictive and happily declare it to you.

Accordingly, we need to do a little carb detox here, Betty. Reducing carbohydrates has been shown to have a direct impact on mortality.[90] Eating a plant-rich, nutrient-dense diet is a way for you to live a longer, healthier life and be around to play with your grandchildren and great grandchildren. You are building a legacy, and I want to help you live the longest life you can, Betty. For your metabolism, that means eating a carbohydrate appropriate diet.

THE ESTIMA DIET: THE FOUNDATIONAL BASIC

An easy, overarching way to think about structuring your

meals and building your plate is by asking yourself these three questions:

Where are the plants?

Where are the proteins?

Where are the fats?

When building out your meal, the plants should make up the majority of the plate (think a bed of sautéed Swiss chard or roasted Brussels sprouts, lightly steamed broccoli, or a pile of spinach). The protein should be about the size of your palm, and the fat, in the form of dressing or marinade, is the fill.

Now keep in mind, this is where a lot of people get tripped up because the fat is going to be the smallest in terms of quantity but has more calories than the other macronutrients combined! Fat has nine calories per gram (abbreviated 9 kcal/g) while carbohydrates and proteins have less than half of that, clocking in at 4 kcal/g. Fat is more calorically dense than proteins or carbohydrates, and therefore we need to be mindful of how much we consume. When you drizzle olive oil on your salad, a little goes a long way.

The caloric breakdown of this first phase of the diet is a 70-20-10 split. Meaning 70 percent of your calories will be from fat, 20 percent of your calories will be from proteins, and 10 percent will be from nutrient-dense carbohydrates.

Here is an example of a typical Estima Diet Protocol:

BREAKFAST: GREEN EGGS AND HAM

Prep Time: five minutes | Cook Time: ten minutes | Serves four

INGREDIENTS

3 oz Canadian Bacon (Pancetta, Bacon, and Smoked Ham are also options)

1 tbsp / 15mL coconut oil

4 large eggs

Pinch of sea salt

Green Hollandaise:

6 Basil Leaves

¼ cup grass fed butter or ghee

1 egg yolk

2 tbsp lemon juice

INSTRUCTIONS:

Preheat oven to 425F

Place bacon on a baking sheet in the oven until crisp (10–15 minutes, depending on your oven)

Meanwhile, make the hollandaise sauce: Pop all ingredients into a blender and blitz until fully blended

Prepare the eggs: For sunny side up, heat coconut oil in a skillet over medium heat and crack eggs into the pan. It takes about 5 minutes for the egg white to be fully cooked through.

Remove eggs from the pan and plate them over the bacon. Drizzle the green hollandaise sauce over top.

Meal Macronutrients Per Serving (1)

Calories 258 kcal

Fat: 23 g

Protein: 10.5 g

Carbohydrate: 1 g

LUNCH: DR. STEPHANIE'S CITRUS CHICKEN WITH GRAVY AND ASPARAGUS

Prep Time: fifteen minutes | Cook Time: 1.5 hours | Serves six

INGREDIENTS:

1 whole chicken

2 lemons

1 orange

1 head of garlic

4 garlic cloves

5 tbsp olive oil

1.5 tbsp Greek or Italian seasoning

1 lb/16 oz asparagus

INSTRUCTIONS:

Preheat the oven to 400F.

Zest the orange and lemon peels in a separate mixing bowl. Quarter the zested orange and lemon. Whisk the orange zest, lemon zest, oil, oregano, and chopped garlic in a medium bowl to blend. Brush some of the juice mixture over the chicken.

Stuff the chicken cavity with the quartered orange, lemon, and garlic halves. Tie the chicken legs together with kitchen string. Season the chicken with salt and pepper.

Place a rack in a large roasting pan. Place the chicken, breast side up, on the rack in the pan. Roast the chicken for one hour, basting occasionally and adding some chicken broth or water to the pan, if necessary, to prevent the pan drippings from burning.

After an hour, flip the chicken, so it is breast side down. Continue roasting the chicken until an instant-read meat thermometer inserted into the innermost part of the thigh registers 170F, basting occasionally with the zest mixture and adding broth to the pan, about forty-five minutes longer. Skin on both sides should be crispy.

Transfer the chicken to a platter. Do not clean the pan.

Place the same roasting pan (with all the drippings) over medium-low heat.

Whisk in any remaining broth and simmer until the sauce is reduced to 1 cup/250 mL, stirring often, about three minutes. Strain into a 2 cup/500 mL glass measuring cup and discard the solids. Serve the chicken with the pan sauce.

About ten minutes before the bird is done, steam the asparagus. Serve alongside your citrus chicken masterpiece.

Meal Macronutrients Per Serving

Calories: 313 kcals

Fat: 21 g

Protein: 29 g

Carbohydrates: 5 g

DINNER: STEAK WITH BEARNAISE SAUCE

Prep Time: five minutes, plus forty minutes to rest before cooking, and five minutes to rest after | Cook Time: ten minutes | Serves: four

INGREDIENTS:

2 T-bone or rib-eye steaks (about 2 lbs/32 oz/908 g total)

1 tbsp sea salt (or to taste)

2 tsp fresh ground black pepper (or to taste)

Melted coconut oil

Butter Bearnaise Sauce:

1 tbsp/15 mL plus 1 cup/250 mL (2 sticks) Unsalted butter

3 tbsp shallots, minced

2 tbsp white wine vinegar

2 large egg yolks

1 tbsp fresh lemon juice

1 tbsp/15 mL fresh tarragon, chopped

INSTRUCTIONS:

Season the steaks with salt and pepper. Let the seasoned steak rest for at least 30 minutes at room temperature.

Meanwhile, prepare the Béarnaise: Melt 1 tbsp butter in a saucepan over medium heat. Add shallots and stir in vinegar. Reduce heat to low, and cook until vinegar is evaporated, 3–4 minutes. Continue cooking shallots, stirring frequently, until tender and translucent, 5 minutes longer. Transfer shallots to a bowl and set aside.

Melt remaining 1 cup/250 mL butter in a saucepan over medium heat and then transfer butter to a bowl to cool.

Combine egg yolks, lemon juice, and 1 tbsp/15 mL water in a blender. Puree mixture until smooth. With blender running, slowly pour in hot butter in a thin stream. Continue blending for 3 minutes. Pour sauce into a medium bowl. Stir in shallot reduction and tarragon and season to taste with salt and pepper.

Preheat a grill pan to high heat.

Melt the coconut oil or lard. Place the marinated steaks on the hot grill and do not move them for about 2 minutes. Use tongs to flip the steaks and grill for 2 more minutes.

Cook 3 more minutes for rare, 4 more minutes for medium-rare, 5 more minutes for medium, 6 to 7 minutes for medium-well, and 8 to 10 minutes for well done.

Remove steaks from the grill and let them rest for at least 5 minutes before cutting into them. Serve with the bearnaise sauce.

Listen to awesome 80s music and enjoy.

Meal Macronutrient Per Serving (1)

Calories: 915 kcals

Fat: 80 g

Protein: 46g

Carbohydrates: 1 g

I also have prepared four weeks' worth of recipes that are a part of The Estima Diet for you. Just head over to www. bettybodybook.com/bonus.

CHOLESTEROL IS ACTUALLY YOUR FAIRY GODMOTHER

Now I understand this statement may be shocking to some, especially those of you who grew up in the low-fat, high-carb diet era. We have been told that fat clogs our arteries, raises cholesterol, and primes us for heart attacks. The thing is, our liver produces upwards of 80 percent of the cholesterol in our bodies. Eighty percent, Betty! That means modulating your dietary cholesterol up or down won't make a major dent in your cholesterol levels.[91] And if you are too aggressive in your cholesterol-lowering efforts, your liver, the wiley smart minx that she is, will start to increase her production of cholesterol to make up for the lack of it in your diet.

On the contrary, it is in the consumption of excess carbo-hydrates where we run into a problem. Excess carbohydrate consumption has been shown to upregulate triglyceride pro-duction and low-density lipoproteins (LDL). These low-density proteins are much more susceptible to oxidative damage and contributing to *atherogenesis*, or the formation of arterial plaquing. The combination of low fat, high carbohydrate con-sumption is one of the major contributing factors to cholesterol issues and pre-diabetes.[92]

I think it is high time we finally sing the praises of cholesterol. It is a necessary structural element in the brain and nervous system, and it is the mother from which all your sex hormones are made! Your progesterone, estrogens, testosterones, and cor-tisol are all synthesized from cholesterol.

This is why I am not a fan of low cholesterol diets over the long term. I think this dietary approach has been a major failure that persists today. In one study of over fifty-two thousand Nor-wegians, researchers found that women with total cholesterol levels below 195 mg/dL had a higher risk of death than women with cholesterol levels above that cut-off.[93] Another study published in the American Journal of Medicine found that people over seventy years of age with total cholesterol levels below 160 mg/dL had twice the risk of death than those with cholesterol levels between 160-199 mg/dL.[94]

Low cholesterol is also associated with an increased risk of disease, especially mental health and brain disorders. Low cholesterol has been associated with premature death from unnatural causes,[95] depression in both men and women,[96] dementia,[97] and Alzheimer's Disease.[98]

So, it isn't necessarily the fat that is plaquing our arteries. It is the overconsumption of carbohydrates (that are often processed) that lead to these dire outcomes.

WHY THE ESTIMA DIET IS MEANT FOR WOMEN

There are a few key differences with this female-focused keto plan when compared to others. Namely:

- Vegetables High in Insoluble Fiber
- Resistant Starches

These two foods are a winning combination for women.

INSOLUBLE FIBER AND RESISTANT STARCHES FOR THE WIN

Not all carbohydrates are created equal, and there is a reason we eat boatloads of vegetables with this plan. Green leafy vegetables like kale, spinach, swiss chard, bok choy, and broccoli, and fermented foods like sauerkraut and kimchi all have an extraordinary amount of insoluble fiber. Insoluble fiber plays an important role in becoming fat adapted and ketogenic.

The fiber found in green leafy vegetables is *insoluble*; it cannot be broken down by gut bacteria to be used for energy. This insoluble fiber will pass through the intestinal tract, cleaning up debris, sopping up excess hormones, and cleaning out the gut like a pipe cleaner. Eating foods high in fiber is also a great way to make stool bulky and softer. Consuming fiber does not affect blood sugar levels, and therefore has a negligible effect on insulin. Effectively, they are carbs that do not count as carbs!

As we mentioned in Chapter 5, resistant starches are carbohydrates that don't *technically* count as carbs because they cannot be broken down in the gut for energy. Instead of being digested for energy, they selectively feed the "good" microbiota in our gut. As these microbiota chow down on the resistant starches, they produce short-chain fatty acids as a by-product of their meal.[99] Of particular importance here is the short-chain fatty acid known as *butyrate*. Butyrate has a whole host of beneficial effects, including decreasing gut permeability.[100]

When the lining of the gut is more permeable, we are more susceptible to developing food allergies, food intolerances, and an immune system on high alert all the time. Having increased permeability of the gut has been associated with almost all proinflammatory conditions, including most autoimmune conditions, fatty liver disease, and heart disease.[101]

Remember, stress is the lynchpin of most lifestyle diseases. One of the primary objectives we must look at in any health protocol is healing the gut. The obvious reason here is a healthy gut makes digesting food a more pleasant and efficient experience.

We all want to eat without gas, bloating, indigestion, or diarrhea. But it is the knock-on positive benefits to our neurology that are of particular long-term importance. The gut has its own nervous system, called the *enteric nervous system*, which has strong communication pathways with the brain and central nervous system. So, when we feed the gut, and it produces butyrate levels that are high, you allow gut healing to occur. And butyrate is a gift that keeps on giving—butyrate helps keep the brain healthy by upping the expression of neurotrophic factors, which is to say that these neurotrophic factors help your brain stay dense with lots of neurons![102]

Consuming resistant starches help in the maintenance of nerve cells that you already have, but also help grow new, healthy nerve cells. In other words—butyrate keeps your brain big and juicy.

MACRONUTRIENTS AND CHOOSING YOUR CALORIES

The most common questions I'm asked are, "How many calories should I start with?" and, "How will I know if I am eating too much or too little?" In this section, we are going to help you determine the daily caloric intake you can start with. I am going to lay out some math, so bear with me, but the overarching guide will be your hunger signals. When you get that familiar pang of hunger, you must ask yourself the following question: am I truly hungry, or am I thirsty, upset, or just bored? Before heading for the fridge, drink a tall glass of water and wait. Because thirst and hunger signals often feel the same, we often mistake thirst for hunger, resulting in our taking in too many calories. You can also ask yourself if you are reaching for food due to an emotional trigger or fatigue.

To determine how many calories you burn every day just to live, otherwise known as the Harris-Benedict equation, plug the appropriate numbers into the following equation:

BMR = (10 × weight in kg) + (6.25 × height in cm) – (5 × age in years) – 161

Now take that number and multiply it based on how active you are:

Lifestyle	Example	Calculation
Sedentary or light activity	Office worker getting little or no exercise	BMR x 1.53
Active or moderately active	Running or exercising one hour daily	BMR x 1.76
Vigorously active	Equivalent of two hours daily, hard labor	BMR x 2.25

This is an estimate of your total caloric expenditure and has an accuracy of +/– 210 calories for women. So, let's say after going through these steps, your number is 2,300 kcals/day. That means eating about 1,800 calories per day is going to put you at a deficit of approximately 500 kcals / day, or 1 pound per week. What I have found in practice and in my online program, The Estima Method, is that most women have a hard time even getting to 1,800 calories because fat is so satiating!

To get your macronutrients to match your caloric intake, I have included a chart with calories and the corresponding macronutrient ratios you should eat in the appendix section of this book.

MACRONUTRIENT CHART MINUS THE MATH

To avoid having to do math, I have taken the initiative to calculate your macronutrient intake for you. I created this chart for reference to build out your 70-20-10 ketosis program, and it will also serve you when you get to cycling keto in Chapter 12.

First, choose your calories based on the equations above, then follow the gram intake of your fats, proteins, and carbohydrates. For example, if you have calculated your calories to be 1,500 kcals, in a 70-20-10 split that would be 117 g of fat, 75 g of protein, and 38 g of carbohydrates. In Chapter 12, when there are weeks where your macros will be 40-40-20, 1,500 calories split would be 67 g of fat, 150 g of protein, and 75 g of carbohydrates.

CALORIES	1300	1400	1500	1600	1700	1800	1900	2000	2100	2200	2300	2400	2500	2600	2700	2800	2900	3000
%	**GRAMS**																	
FAT																		
70%	101	109	117	124	132	140	148	156	163	171	179	187	194	202	210	218	226	253
65%	94	101	108	116	123	130	137	144	152	159	166	173	181	188	195	202	209	217
60%	87	93	100	107	113	120	127	133	140	147	153	160	167	173	180	187	193	200
55%	79	86	92	98	104	110	116	122	128	134	141	147	153	159	165	171	177	183
50%	72	78	83	89	94	100	106	111	117	122	128	133	139	144	150	156	161	167
45%	65	70	75	80	85	90	95	100	105	110	115	120	125	130	135	140	145	150
40%	58	62	67	71	76	80	84	89	93	98	102	107	111	116	120	124	129	133
PROTEIN																		
40%	130	140	150	160	170	180	190	200	210	220	230	240	250	260	270	280	290	300
35%	114	123	131	140	149	158	166	175	184	193	201	210	219	228	236	245	254	263
30%	98	105	113	120	128	135	143	150	158	165	173	180	188	195	203	210	218	225
25%	81	88	94	100	106	113	119	125	131	138	144	150	156	163	169	175	181	188
20%	65	70	75	80	85	90	95	100	105	110	115	120	125	130	135	140	145	150
CARBS																		
20%	65	70	75	80	85	90	95	100	105	110	115	120	125	130	135	140	145	150
15%	49	53	56	60	64	68	71	75	79	83	86	90	94	98	101	105	109	113
10%	33	35	38	40	43	45	50	53	55	58	60	63	65	68	70	73	75	78
5%	16	18	19	20	21	23	24	25	26	28	29	30	31	33	34	35	36	38

KETO FLU AND PEEING: A FEW OBSERVATIONS FROM THE FIRST TWO WEEKS

As you are about to jump into four weeks of ketosis, be fore-warned—the first two weeks can be tough to navigate as your body depletes its carbohydrate stores and moves toward fat burning. For some, this is a walk in the park, and for others, it can feel like you've been hit by a mack truck if you are not prepared.

First, you will quickly notice you are taking lots of trips to the bathroom to pee. This is because carbohydrates are typically stored with three to four molecules of water. So, as we work through and use up our carbohydrate stores, we also shed water retention.

Then, slowly, around the end of the first week, you might begin to feel a little "off." The symptoms can begin to mimic a mild to moderate flu: headaches, brain fog, muscle aches, and even nausea. Some women also notice their skin gets worse, or their breath gets bad. Both of these occurrences are temporary. I've even had clients who suffer from frequent UTIs feel like these get kicked up a notch, too.

These symptoms don't happen with everyone, but if they occur with you, know it is all temporary. Your body is switching metabolic gears and going through a sugar detox. It's normal for there to be a worsening of some symptoms as the body is expunging sugars. In my observation, this discomfort typically lasts for two to three days, and then it is gone. One of the best ways to get through this detox is by ensuring you are drinking a lot of water and taking electrolytes. Remember, as you use up carbohydrates, you are also getting rid of water. And with the water loss, so go your essential electrolytes. A simple way to fix this is to put a pinch of salt in an eight-ounce glass of water.

The reason you feel so crappy is your body is transitioning into fat burning. When I entered nutritional ketosis for the first time, I felt like I had just completed a marathon and had zero energy. Given my years of sugar-coffee and the terrible diet from my college years, activating my fat burning was like oiling the gears of a bike that had been sitting in a shed for twenty years. I walked into my home after a day of seeing patients and face-planted on the bed. It was awful, and rightly so. It was the first time I burned fat as my main energy source, and my body did its best to keep up and adapt. After about a week, I was on the other side of bliss. All the flu-like symptoms were gone, my mind was clear, and I had boundless energy. I felt almost high! My brain was sharp, my sleep was deep, and most joyously, I was happy.

WHEN TO MOVE ON FROM 100 PERCENT KETOSIS

Pinkie promise me that you will redo the quizzes, trackers, and sheets at the end of each month, no matter how many cycles of The Estima Diet you have completed. This is because what you measure, you manage. It is so easy to forget where you started, and how much progress you have made! Do you remember how your energy levels were three months ago? I'd wager that you may have a faint idea but can't come up with specifics. The monthly testing will give you a chance to see your progress and how far you've come, what tweaks you need to make next month, and how you will continue through this healing journey.

With that in mind, if you have found your weight loss plateauing after several cycles of The Estima Diet, it may be time to move onto the next phase of this program, which is a cyclical ketogenic approach. In Chapter 9, I outline cycling keto and how to pair it with your menstrual cycle. If you are menopausal,

I also recommend moving to this type of cyclical ketogenic plan long-term.

As I mentioned at the beginning of this chapter, women are not meant to be in ketosis forever. More importantly, as we age, we want to think about developing and maintaining muscle, and we can do this through exercise (which we'll discuss in Chapter 13) and nutrition. As you will see in Chapter 9, there will be weeks where you will eat more protein, and weeks where you will eat more carbs.

Ketosis was once an ancient back up—an energetic insurance policy for when food was sparse. Drawing on our natural fat reserves, it is designed to supply our body and brain with the energy it needs without sacrificing functional tissue like muscle. But we can't be in ketosis forever. We can use this ancient system to our advantage to achieve our weight and metabolic goals, but we also want to attune our cyclical needs to balance our hormones over the long term.

THE ESTIMA DIET: LABS

One of the greatest things about the ketogenic diet is that it is the only diet that has a biomarker, ketone bodies, to tell you how well you are doing on the diet. At a minimum, to be considered in ketosis, we want blood ketone levels to be at least 0.5 mmol/L, which can easily be measured using a blood ketone monitor. This method of measurement is the most accurate and can get expensive quickly with strips costing around one dollar per use. This can add up over time. Other alternatives to measure your ketone levels are a breath analyzer (I personally use the Keyto breath monitor and have found it to track well when compared to blood readings) or urine strips. Urine strips are by far the most economical and can be purchased on Amazon.

I wanted to include this section on monitoring your lipid levels because while 80 to 90 percent of people will do wonderfully on this diet, there is a small percentage of people who do poorly with fats, specifically saturated fats, in their diet. These are known as hyper responders to the ketogenic diet. If this is you, I want to give you the tools to understand and monitor your lipids, and options to modify the diet.

If you have a familial history of wacky lipids, heart attacks, and cardiovascular disease, I strongly suggest monitoring the labs below with your primary doctor or cardiologist. Research has shown over and again that a low carb, high fat diet tends to improve cholesterol, and reduces your risk of cardiovascular disease. It improves all the ratios listed above and lowers tri-glycerides. Now, it is also true that some of us have a longer journey to healthy lipid levels than others. This is especially true if you have experienced chronic low-grade stress for a number of years. Stress is such a cranky bitch, and she just shows up everywhere, including your labs!

Keep in mind, this type of stress often causes some degree of insulin insensitivity. When looking at this in the context of cho-lesterol, stress can also increase your total cholesterol number. As long as you pinky promise to stick to the diet and see it through, this spike in cholesterol is OK if it is for a short amount of time. I always recommend giving yourself six months to see an accurate picture of your metabolic and lipid changes. Otherwise, you might quit before your body has a chance to catch up and adapt.

When you lose weight quickly (which often happens in the first month of this diet), your fat cells spill out their stored triglycerides and cholesterol into the bloodstream, and your liver needs to up her game in clearing them out. As your weight loss slows, your liver has a chance to catch up and regulate everything. However, an underactive thyroid can also temporarily increase the number of LDLs in the blood. This is because the active form of thyroid hormone, T3, plays a central role in activating the LDL receptors on our cells. If your liver is working overtime to clear out the triglycerides and cholesterol from your weight loss, you may also find her conversion of T4 (our inactive thyroid hormone) to T3 (our active thyroid hormone) is slower, too.

Now, what if you've waited six months and your lipids are still wacky? It likely means you are a hyper-responder; someone whose lipid profile gets worse with saturated fats in their diet. In other words, eating a diet with lots of saturated fat is not good for you in the long run. In this scenario, there are a couple of choices you can make. You can quit keto altogether (usually a very unpopular option, but it is still an option), or you can change the type of fat you consume by removing as much saturated fats as you can and instead consuming primarily monounsaturated and polyunsaturated fats. This means limiting red meat and animal fats, and making your source of fats primarily olive oil, nuts, and seeds. This is often the simplest and most popular option, and you can retest your lipid levels again in a few months. The important point here is that you have options.

Even today, lipid and cholesterol management are an ongoing area of debate. Lipid metabolism is incredibly complicated—context and personal and familial history really matter here. What I can tell you for sure is that looking at your total cholesterol number on a lab report is essentially meaningless without the context of HDL, LDL, and the other markers I have listed below.

Total cholesterol: 180–250 (but I'm OK with up to 300 if other ratios are good)

HDL: 50–80 mg/dL

LDL(c): less than 100 mg/dL

LDL(p): under 1000

Triglycerides: less than 100 mg/dL

Lp(a): less than 10 mg/dL*

HbA1C: 5.1 or under

LDL to HDL ratio: 3:1 ratio at the minimum, and 2:1 is ideal

Fasting glucose: 85 mg/dL or under

Non-HDL: Total Cholesterol – HDL. What is cool about this simple calculation is it is highly correlated with your LDL particle number. Meaning if this number is good, it suggests your LDL(p) will likely be good also.

Triglyceride to HDL ratio: 2:1 at a minimum, 1:1 or higher HDL than triglycerides are optimal

*Lp(a) is Lipoprotein a, low-density lipoprotein that has been identified as a risk factor for atherosclerosis, coronary artery disease and stroke

I also like to see contextually fasting glucose paired with a two-hour post-prandial glucose challenge to see how efficiently insulin brings glucose into the cells.

The other biomarker I see that is quickly becoming the marker of choice is Coronary Artery Calcium Score (CAC). This is a measure of how much calcium and calcification exists in the arterial wall. This is a strong marker for cardiovascular risk because, as a plaque progresses, it calcifies. The CAC is like an X-ray for your arteries. Under the age of forty, we expect your CAC score to be zero, meaning there is zero calcification in the arteries. The best-case scenario is for you to be as close to zero as possible, but again, context, including your age and family history, is extremely important here.

WHAT YOU CAN DO THIS WEEK

Clean out your pantry of processed chips, crackers, cookies, and carbohydrates that are no-no's during ketosis. Take a before and after picture of your pantry and tag me on Instagram!

Repeat the twenty-eight-day cycle as many times as you'd like to continue losing weight, or until you plateau. I recommend you repeat this cycle at least three times.

Once you have calculated your caloric intake, structure your macronutrients using the chart in this chapter.

Start using salt or an electrolyte blend in water on a daily basis if you experience lethargy, muscle aches, or headaches (and know this is temporary!).

Head over to www.bettybodybook.com/bonus to download the free Four-Week Meal Plan.

CHAPTER 9

KETO CYCLING FOR ALL WOMEN

When I first developed The Estima Diet, it was a monumental success. As thousands of women did the diet and thousands of pounds were lost, eventually, the question in our community became, "What's next, Doc? Am I never going to eat carbs again?"

I went back to the lab, both with myself and my clients, to develop a long-term protocol to follow once pure ketosis was finished. It had to be a protocol that was complimentary to female physiology and took into consideration our changing hormonal environment and common dietary challenges like cravings. While cycling in and out of ketosis is not a new concept, how it fits into the body of work I have created is to sync it with your menstrual cycle. And if you are in menopause or do not have a menstrual cycle, you'll follow a higher protein version of this protocol.

Regardless of menstrual status, once fat adaptation has been achieved (from your work in Chapter 8), it is highly beneficial to cycle weekly fats, proteins, and carbohydrates. If you are still in your reproductive years, including perimenopause, this will serve two functions. First—you will be eating in harmony with the ever-changing hormonal milieu of your cycle (if you recall from Chapter 3, we are different every single day of the month!), which will support your changing energy, moods, and sleep. Second, it will help you maintain the weight loss achieved from pure ketosis. It will also support your exercise routine and compliment and amplify your body composition.

If you are menopausal, you should still be keto cycling. Women in menopause tend to become more insulin resistant, meaning that eating high amounts of carbohydrates will often lead to blood sugar spikes. We also tend to lose muscle mass as we age if we are not taking precautions both in our diet and at the gym, so it will still be necessary to cycle up proteins throughout the month. Cycling is also a way to avoid boredom, mix up your diet, try new vegetables and recipes, and experiment.

This chapter is best to begin after you've completed at least three cycles of ketosis as outlined in Chapter 8. If you notice your weight loss and other improvements begin to taper off, it is time to switch to the keto cycling outlined in this chapter. This will help maintain your results and honor your natural rhythms over the long term. If you still have more weight to lose despite going through three months of the Estima Diet, skip to Chapter 10 for a deep dive and twelve-week plan to integrate more fasting into your routine. You may also want to visit Chapters 4 and 5 to ensure you are removing environmental toxins like plastics and household cleaners that may be causing inflammation and weight-loss resistance.

PLAYING THE LONG GAME AND AN EXERCISE IN FORGIVENESS

As much as we might resist it, our hormonal fluctuations, not our willpower (or worthiness), are running the show. The more you resist, the more your hormones will push back, driving toward what they need: more calories to help thicken and develop the endometrial lining. You cannot control your cravings through sheer willpower—just like you are not able to voluntarily control your heartbeat or the production of cellular energy. If you find yourself getting hungry the week before your period, it isn't because you cannot control your cravings. It is because your body is using up calories at an accelerated rate and needs more from you.

Most women make the mistake of attempting to eat the same way all through the month. I did this, too, even in my early days of playing with ketosis. I used to be so scared of being knocked out of ketosis that I fought my body to continue carbohydrate restriction, including the week right before my period when my body needed carbohydrates the most. But I write this with the intention of speeding up your learning curve, so you do not make the same mistakes I did. The simple fact is, the hormonal composition of my body and your body are different every single day of the month.

I began collecting data about my cycle. I would track my body temperature, logging in when my period started and finished on an app, how I felt every day, bowel movements, skin (Oily? Breaking out? Dry?) and what foods I was craving. I began, like the mad scientist I am, an unofficial n=1 experiment. My hypothesis was if I changed the ratios of the diet throughout the month it would help to alleviate my anxiety, reduce cravings, and sustain weight loss even when I was not in a state of ketosis. I gave myself objective quizzes like the Cohen Perceived Stress Scale and took it throughout the month. I have included a copy of the quiz in the appendix section. After tweaking and playing with my eating habits for several months, a few distinct patterns emerged.

First, it became apparent that it was much easier to stick to a keto-genic diet during the first two weeks of my cycle, but if I pushed too hard in the last two weeks, and in particular week four, everything would fall apart and I would eat all the cheese and crackers in sight.

In the luteal phase of my cycle, I noticed that I felt more inflamed, and craved more of everything: carbohydrates, pro-teins, and fat overall. This Betty wanted more calories. If I didn't up my caloric intake in week four, I experienced more sleep disturbances, moodiness, anxiety, and stress.

After months of data collection, I started modifying the nutri-tional composition of my diet. I changed up the type of fasting I did throughout the month, making my fasts shorter and less frequent in the luteal phase. I also began increasing protein in weeks two and four of my cycle. That seemed to help with my satiety, exercise recovery, and it also squashed cravings.

And when I finally realized carbs were not the enemy and added in more strategic carbohydrates in weeks three and four, like more leafy green vegetables and resistant starches, the wild beastess within was satisfied and tamed. I was happy, sleep-ing better, and shocker of shockers, had less cravings in week four. Instead of caving to the cravings and going on a carb tear, when I upped my calories with selective veggies, it all went away. My stress scores continued to decline over several months of tracking.

I expanded my n=1 and brought this to my female patients. Same results. And the great news: my ladies in perimenopause and menopause also reaped the benefits of keto cycling, even if they didn't have a period anymore.

I reckon this is so successful for women of all ages because cycling and altering the nutrient composition of the diet will continue to sensitize our muscle cells to protein, reduce cravings, provide a recovery week (in terms of higher carbohydrates), improve our neurotransmitter levels, and improve insulin sensitivity as we age. Irrespective of menstrual status, cycling macronutrients throughout the month is a way to maintain weight loss, improve our moods, and consistently make lean muscle mass gains.

KETO CYCLING
BLEED WEEK / WEEK ONE

As we discussed in Chapter 3, this is the week where all your reproductive hormones go on a mini-vacation. The only one who is holding down the fort is FSH (Follicular Stimulating Hormone) as her primary job is to drive one follicle to maturation and eventually release an egg. From a metabolic perspective, your period week is when your body can better tolerate a low-carbohydrate, or keto diet. This is a time where we can take advantage of a female-appropriate keto diet. In other words, this is one of the best times of the month to comfortably eat a low carb, moderate protein, and high-fat diet as described in Chapter 8. This is because progesterone (a potent stimulant of your appetite) is at its lowest this week, so it is much easier to go low to no carb. Sometimes, the first few days of your period can leave you feeling sluggish and tired, and if that's the case, you can slowly ease into the 70-20-10 protocol after taking the first few days of your period off.

If you have crossed into the golden land of menopause, label this week as week one of your month and adhere to the Estima Protocol outlined in Chapter 8. The macronutrient composition here is 70 percent fat, 20 percent protein, and 10 percent carbohydrates. You can use the macronutrient chart in Chapter 8 to figure out exactly how many grams of fats, proteins, and carbohydrates you will eat this week. Choosing leafy green vegetables will keep your bowel movements singing your praises, and you will avoid rapid increases in blood sugar that come from simple or processed carbohydrates.

BEFORE OVULATION / WEEK TWO

You want to cycle up protein this week, whether you are in menopause or still have your period. If you recall from Chapter 3, testosterone is peaking in women with a cycle this week, so we want to profit from this rise by increasing protein in our diet. For menopausal women who do not have this testosterone rise, it is important to change this week's protein composition to create and maintain muscle mass. The more muscle mass we have, the more testosterone we produce. Testosterone is involved in maintaining lean muscle mass and driving something called *muscle protein synthesis*. By increasing our protein consumption this week, we can amplify muscle protein synthesis.

There are two main ways we can increase muscle growth:

- Through our diet (chemically)
- Through exercise (mechanically)

The key to driving muscle protein synthesis is the consumption of an essential amino acid called leucine. This is a branch chain amino acid that is found abundantly in chicken, meat, eggs, and fish. Leucine is the forewoman that gets muscle protein synthesis started. Multiple studies all suggest about 2.5 g of leucine are required to get the gears turning on muscle protein synthesis.[103]

Practically speaking, this equates to a minimum of 20–25 g of whey or animal protein, or approximately 40 g of soy protein. Now, it is worth stating the obvious here: if you are deriving your protein from vegetarian sources like soy, rice, or peas, you need to consume *more* calories to start the wheels turning for muscle protein synthesis than you would if you consumed whey protein. Animal-derived sources of protein give you more bang for your buck than plant-derived protein sources.

Now, that is not to say you cannot use vegetarian protein sources. Of course, you can, but bear in mind you will need to consume more calories to get the same amount of leucine to get the job done. Let's do some simple math. Let us compare 25 g of whey protein, which yields about 2.5 g of leucine with 40 g of soy protein, which also yields 2.5 g of leucine. Both the 25 g of whey and the 40 g of soy are going to get that forewoman, leucine, to drive muscle protein synthesis, but consider the caloric difference:

25 g of whey protein

25 g * 4 kcal/g = 100 kcals

40 g of soy protein

40 g * 4 kcal/g = 160 kcals

It is important to continue driving muscle protein synthesis as efficiently as we can as we age. As women age, we naturally lose muscle and bone density. To make matters worse, as we get older, a phenomenon known as *anabolic resistance* begins to set in.[104] What this means is the muscle tissue becomes less and less sensitive to leucine, so we need *more* of it to drive that precious muscle protein synthesis. If we are constantly getting our protein from vegetarian sources, it will require a continuous increase in calories for muscle protein synthesis to occur. While weight management is far more than just calories in versus calories out, constantly elevated caloric consumption will lead to weight gain, and an undoing of all the good work you put in to lose the weight in the first place.

This anabolic resistance that happens as we age is thought to be one of the underlying causal factors in sarcopenic obesity and osteoporosis.[105] *Sarcopenic obesity* is a type of obesity caused by a loss of muscle mass, along with fatty infiltration of the muscle tissue. This leaves women with less muscle tissue, and the quality of the remaining muscle tissue is marbled with fat. Our bones and our muscles are best friends, and what happens to one happens to the other. Loss of muscle mass is directly related to loss of bone density, and vice versa.

My solution to this decrease in protein sensitivity as we age is to cycle protein while we have a menstrual cycle, and to continue this practice through menopause. This will capitalize on our ability to synthesize muscle as testosterone peaks in our reproductive years and will help counter the increased nitrogen utilization in the week before your period. Protein consumption is also highly satiating, so you will feel fuller when your body naturally craves more calories in the week leading up to your period.

When cycling up protein, I reduce fat intake. I generally like to change my macronutrients up in the following way: 40 percent fat, 40 percent protein, 20 percent carbohydrates. If you are using this higher protein macronutrient composition and taking in 1500 kcals of energy per day, 40 percent is about 150 g of high quality (high leucine) protein. Spreading that over three meals, it works out to 50 grams of protein per meal.

A sample day with this macronutrient breakdown might look like this:

POST WORKOUT RECOVERY SHAKE

1 scoop whey protein with water

1 oz steel cut oats or sugar-free rice puff cereal

Shake Macronutrients Per Serving (1)

Calories: 185 kcals

Fat: 2 g

Protein: 28 g

Carbohydrates: 13 g

BREAKFAST—METABOLIC SHAKE

INGREDIENTS

¾ cup unsweetened coconut milk (or almond milk)

1/3 cup frozen blueberries

1 scoop whey protein powder

10 mL MCT Oil

1 cup of water

Blend all ingredients and drink immediately.

Shake Macronutrients Per Serving (1)

Calories: 275 kcals

Fat: 14 g

Protein: 24 g

Carbohydrates: 12 g

LUNCH—CHICKEN WITH MANGO SALSA

INGREDIENTS

4 oz boneless, skinless chicken breast

3 oz mango, chopped

3 oz cucumber, chopped

2 tsp red onion diced

2 tbsp lime juice

1 tbsp extra virgin olive oil

Salt and pepper

INSTRUCTIONS

Combine the mango, cucumber, red onion, and lime juice and mix well.

Season with salt and pepper to taste.

Meanwhile, grill or bake the chicken breast. Slice into strips and plate over the mango salsa.

Macronutrients Per Serving (1)

Calories: 390 kcal

Fat: 19 g

Protein: 37 g

Carbohydrates: 16 g

DINNER—WILD BAKED SALMON
WITH CABBAGE SLAW

INGREDIENTS

5 oz wild-caught salmon

4 oz red cabbage, thinly sliced

2 oz carrots, grated

½ oz dried cranberries

2 walnuts

10 mL mayonnaise

10 mL raw honey

10 mL apple cider vinegar

INSTRUCTIONS

Preheat oven to 425F. Place salmon on a tray with parchment paper and bake for 18–20 minutes.

Meanwhile, combine the rest of the ingredients (red cabbage, carrots, cranberries, walnuts, mayo, raw honey and apple cider vinegar) into a bowl and stir well.

Macronutrients Per Serving (1)

Calories: 522 kcals

Fat: 24 g

Protein: 40 g

Carbohydrates: 33 g

I've created a four-week keto cycling meal plan with recipes and nutritional breakdown at www.bettybodybook.com/bonus.

AFTER OVULATION / WEEK THREE

This week is a great time to return to the classic Estima Protocol (high fat / low carb) with a few considerations. In addition to the 70 percent fat, 20 percent protein, 10 percent carbohydrate macronutrient composition, consider adding elements that will help heal the gut and reduce cravings. Specifically, I advise consuming resistant starches every other day (such as green banana flour, green plantain flour, or raw potato starch). Another wonderful way to help reduce cravings is a big increase in leafy green vegetables like kale, Swiss chard, arugula, and spinach. Our bodies are starting to drive up development of the endometrial lining, so adding supplements like magnesium and a full spectrum B vitamin are in order here.

These practices will all help the integrity of the gut and support the nutritional needs of our reproductive cycle. We often forget that when it comes to weight loss, the most important relationship is between your gut and your brain. Remember that resistant starches help to blunt cravings, excess hunger, and control for fluctuations in blood sugar when we eat carbohydrates. They are a natural carbohydrate blocker.

BEFORE YOUR PERIOD / WEEK FOUR

In week four, we want to return to a higher protein, higher carbohydrate composition of the diet. Similar to week two, we will follow a higher protein intake week, approximating 40 percent fat, 40 percent protein, and 20 percent carbohydrates. There are several benefits of adopting this style of eating this week.

First, if you're menopausal, eating this way will continue to support muscle protein synthesis, and protein helps with satiety (feeling full). For women who still have a cycle, the increase in complex carbohydrates will replenish the nutrients and minerals depleted this week, as well as curb your sweet tooth cravings. The increase in strategic carbohydrates, like more green vegetables, will provide your body with the fiber it needs to have regular bowel movements, and this week is notorious for a slow-down in gut motility under the influence of progesterone.

For women who are still cycling, we also want to increase our total caloric intake by 10–15 percent. This is because we are now using all types of energy (carbs, proteins, and fats) at a higher rate to build the endometrium. Now, I know an increase in calorie consumption is going to feel radical, and even a little uncomfortable, especially if you grew up hearing that eating less and exercising more is the solution for weight loss. Let me assure you, the increase in calories is because you *need* them and will be using them all up.

Eating more calories is necessary to honor what is required of your cells this week. Your ovaries and entire reproductive system are working at a frenzied pace right now.[106] The endometrial lining is thickening by the hour, diligently building up its architecture in the event of the reception of a fertilized egg. Your progesterone ascends to its peak in this week, hoping to continue on into pregnancy. If you keep your calories the same as you normally do, you will experience moodiness, low energy, sleep disturbances, headaches, and other common symptoms of someone who is calorie restricting.

And pssst, by the way...I'm not suggesting you clear out an ice cream parlor or eat the entire block of cheese. I'm suggesting a 10 to 15 percent increase in calories. If you are consuming 1,500 kcals during the other three weeks of your cycle, this week you increase by 150 kcals to 225 kcals. That might be one protein bar, or an extra ounce of meat on your plate at each meal. This week, like any other, is a time to be strategic, understand what is going on in your body, and honor the process—the unique process of potentially creating a life. Life needs calories. By increasing calories, and cutting the anxiety about feeding yourself more, you begin to honor, and dare I say, *nourish* more of you.

WHAT YOU CAN DO THIS WEEK

Download the meal plans I have prepared for you at www. bettybodybook.com/bonus.

Figure out where you are in your cycle and begin to follow the nutrient breakdown specific to that week. If you are on your period, follow The Classic Estima Protocol: 70 percent fat, 20 percent protein, 10 percent carbohydrates. The week before ovulation, increase both protein and carbohydrates to take advantage of testosterone's peak in the cycle. This will drive muscle protein synthesis and contribute to building lean muscle mass. My recommendation for macronutrient design is 40 percent fat, 40 percent protein, and 20 percent carbohydrates.

If you have just ovulated, return to the Estima Diet that we call for in week one: 70 percent fat, 20 percent protein, 10 percent carbohydrates, with consideration for the requirements of the luteal phase. Consume resistant starches every other day to curb cravings, blunt the hunger response, and proactively reduce inflammation. And if you are just about to have your period, increase your proteins, carbohydrates, and total calories by 10–15 percent.

If you are menopausal, follow the cycle of alternating weeks of higher protein and then higher fat. Label this week as "week one" and follow a 70-20-10 ketogenic program. Next week, increase your protein intake and decrease your fat so that you are consuming 40 percent fat, 40 percent protein, and 20 percent carbohydrate. It's also ideal to lift heavier weights this week (which we will discuss in Chapter 13). In week three, return to 70-20-10, followed by another high protein week in week four. This will help improve insulin sensitivity, satiety, and muscle sensitivity to protein.

CHAPTER 10

FASTING

Fasting is where we need to honor our unique biology as women. The dialogue is often that fasting can be applied equally to men and women, as if there are no differences between us. I have seen too many experts encourage multi-day water fasts without any regard for a woman's unique biology, menstrual status, and hormonal landscape. We have a complex hormonal landscape that is distinct from men, and as such, there is an opportunity for things to go awry if we ignore that fact. Woman are physiologically more complex.

As a woman, if you fast without consideration for your biology, some literature suggests you are likely going to mess up your ovaries, reproductive capacity, sleep cycles, and anxiety.[107] And listen. I get how frustrating it is to hear that, Betty. I know all too well that a Type A woman wants to put her head down and push through whatever ail, pain, or signal her body tells her to get the job done. I am one of those women!

Even though the physiological benefits of fasting are astounding, everything from weight loss, improved lipid profiles, mental clarity, better sleep, improved fertility to better digestion, it is not always the same for women. It continues to be an ongoing struggle to find data specific to non-obese females who want to fast. The data surrounding women who are of a healthier weight or looking to shed between five to twenty-five pounds is sparse and hard to find. In fact, the few studies that exist do show a distinct phenotypic difference in the effects of fasting for men and women who are not obese.

This is where the intersection of information from the literature and application as a clinician meet. If the data is not clear from the literature, a clinician must take what does exist and pair it with her clinical experience and understanding of female biology. Then, she comes up with a plan, evaluates its effectiveness, and tweaks where necessary. I have been in the "lab" (my private practice) for several years now, and clear patterns have emerged. What follows is a discussion of my clinical observations and personal experiences as a woman. I will explain how fasting is, indeed, different for us.

SHRINKING OVARIES

A particular study creates one of the strongest arguments for ditching calorie restriction as a long-term diet strategy for women. This study[108] looked at the effects of rodents undergoing either 20 percent CR (caloric restriction), 40 percent CR and Intermittent Fasting (IF), or high-fat, high-glucose meals. After six months, females who restricted their calories by 40 percent became abnormally thin and weak, lost their ability to menstruate, and demonstrated enlargement of their adrenal glands alongside a heightened stress response, with a fourfold increase in sleep disturbances.

The males had a completely different outcome. Blurg. Of course, they did! The males in the 40 percent group did not appear emaciated, did not have any changes to their reproductive organs, and did not show a heightened stress response.

Women who fast for long periods of time (and when I say long, I am referring to a period of time longer than twenty-four hours) report many more sleep disturbances, both in falling asleep and the maintenance of sleep.

In my practice, women reported that while attempting longer fasts, they often had trouble falling asleep and woke up several times. And in my case, I had bizarre dreams of eating food. Peculiarly, this happens to me each and every time I undergo a fast longer than twenty-four hours in length. When we look at this with an evolutionary lens, it is likely that this sleep disturbance from caloric scarcity would cause us to forage a larger area to find more food. This behavior could lead to maximizing the probability of survival during periods of food scarcity.

As we discussed in Chapter 2, women today already have a tendency towards sympathetic dominance (our stressed-out, fight or flight response) because of our biology. This is to say we are much more likely to be in a state of chronic low-grade stress from physical, chemical, and emotional stressors that remain unresolved in our nervous system. Think of the physical stress of pregnancy, labor, and delivery, the nutritional demands of breastfeeding, the lack of attention to our diets, and the emotional torture that sleep deprivation can impart.

For the most part, in our society, caregiving of our little ones falls primarily on the mother. She often starts her marathon into motherhood tired and physically exhausted from labor and delivery. There is a true meaning behind the term, "It takes a village to raise a child." That is how we used to do it. There were two to three generations of mothers, aunts, and older children willing and able to help out. Now, we live in single-dwelling homes, many times living far away from our parents in a state of bewilderment, exhaustion, and worry.

HOW DO WOMEN FAST THEN?

Although sleep disturbances, cyclical disturbances, and stress have often been reported to me from healthy women engaging in prolonged caloric restriction or fasting, not all hope is lost.

You still can and should fast. I like to think of fasting as having three distinct levers, all of which can be pulled depending on your goals. They can be aggressive when a lot of weight loss is required or if you have PCOS and desperately want to get your period back to normal. They can be gentler for when we enter our luteal phase and still want to reap some benefits but not go full tilt. The three levers you can pull are the type, frequency, and length of fast.

TYPE OF FASTS
NON-CALORIC LIQUID FASTS

A non-caloric liquid fast is simply a fast with no calories. Water, herbal tea, and black coffee are the only liquids that make the cut. It can be practiced in a daily time-restricted eating model, as well as in an extended fast.

This is the most aggressive type of fast and typically the most challenging for women, especially those with a healthy body weight. I typically reserve this kind of fasting for women who are obese and have a lot of weight to lose, or for women with high fasting glucose levels. If you are obese or morbidly obese, periodic water fasting can be an effective tool for shedding excess adipose tissue and normalizing physiology.

For women who are obese and have been diagnosed with poly-cystic ovarian syndrome (PCOS), this is a very useful type of fasting to help normalize hormone levels. Back in Chapter 4, we discussed hormonal issues around high testosterone. A woman who is having issues with high testosterone may find her weight gain to look similar to the pattern associated with men. That is to say, weight accumulates in the belly region. This woman typically has high insulin levels, which will also increase free circulating testosterone levels. A water fast will help to bring down insulin levels, usually within the first twelve hours of the fast.[109]

CALORIC LIQUID FASTS

Caloric liquid fasting is not technically a pure fast, because during the "fast" you are consuming foods with calories such as bone broth or coffee and tea with fat or collagen in it. A caloric liquid fast is a great tool to use for healing and repairing the gut, mainly because this type of fasting is reparative to the gut lining, and it is easier for your gut to absorb nutrients in liquid form. You are what you *absorb* more so than what you *eat*.

Caloric liquid fasts are also great because they help facilitate better absorption of nutrients. Because the food is liquid, the digestive system does not work as hard to break down and absorb food. When looking at the wear and tear of the gut over time, much of the damage happens at the innermost layer, which is made up of epithelial cells.[110] These specialized cells are necessary for secretion (to break down foods) and absorption (to derive nutrients from foods). Regular caloric fasting may be particularly useful for repairing your gut if you experience symptoms associated with gut health issues like leaky gut, low energy and moodiness, chronic fatigue, allergies, arthritis, food sensitivities, eczema, psoriasis, and recurring lung infections.

Caloric liquid fasts, especially those that are pure bone broth, are so helpful for healing the gut. Bone broth is rich in glutamine, an amino acid that intestinal epithelial cells gobble up and use for energy.[111] Additionally, the collagen and gelatin help to strengthen the mucosal layer in the gut. Gelatin absorbs water and helps to keep aggressive bacteria and other microbes from passing through the intestinal wall.

For your skeleton, which is the structural foundation of your body, bone broth provides the perfect ingredients for building badass strong bones:

- Calcium
- Phosphorus
- Amino acids
- Red and yellow marrow

Bone broth is also excellent for your joints, tendons, and ligaments because of a little ditty called Glycosaminoglycan (or GAGs for short), which is integral for connective tissue and synovial fluid.[112] GAGs allow for proper joint lubrication and pliability. This means they allow for one bone that makes up part of a joint to glide across the other without pain (hello full and painless range of motion!).

A caloric liquid fast is probably one of my favorite fasts for women. It allows for repair of the gut, and a bump up in lubrication of the joints. Both of which, gut issues and joint issues, I have often found to be common in women in their forties and beyond.

You can make your own bone broth by reserving bones from chicken or going to your local butcher and asking for long bones like femurs. Soak the bones in vinegar for at least half an hour before cooking. Then throw in vegetables of your choice—I usually toss in onions, carrots, celery, garlic, and tomatoes, and let it simmer in my slow cooker for a few days. Drain the vegetables, bones, and the layer of fat that accumulates at the top, and your broth is ready to drink or serve as a stock for future meals.

If making broth is not your thing, you can buy from companies like Kettle and Fire. Their broth is stocked in my pantry when I need it and haven't had time to prepare my own.

LENGTH OF FAST

The next option in building out what type of fast works best for you is to alter the length of your fast. The good news is, you already fast every single night when you are sleeping. Your goal then, Betty, should you choose to accept it, is to build your fasting tolerance by *slowly* increasing the hours in which you are fasting on either side of your sleep schedule. The first recommendation is to start with a time-restricted eating regimen of a twelve-hour fast, and a twelve-hour eating window. Meaning, you eat your food within twelve hours, and fast for the rest of the day and night. Since we already sleep (and fast) for eight hours, this simply means extending your fast on either end of your sleep.

If you have your first bite of food at seven o'clock in the morning, you should aim to consume all your calories before seven o'clock in the evening. Doable, right? If you are new to fasting, this should be practiced and mastered for fourteen consecutive days (two weeks) before moving on to the next step.

A TWELVE-WEEK FASTING PROTOCOL
TIME RESTRICTED EATING WITH A NIGHT LIMITER

Once you have mastered the twelve-hour fast and refeed rhythm, the next step is to coordinate eating so that you finish your food three hours before bedtime. This is primarily because we want the stomach to fully empty so it can sync with our sleep and wake cycles, known as our circadian rhythms. We are creatures of habit, and we maintain those habits via circadian rhythms.[113]

The communication between various clocks in our body and the master clock in our brain helps regulate our natural sleep and wake cycles.[114] One of the best ways to sync your central and peripheral clocks is to stop eating after seven o'clock in the evening. As I taught you in Chapter 6, allowing the stomach several hours to empty food (while you are upright) will correct for mixed messages between your brain and body. Or, as a more general rule of thumb, stop eating three to four hours before bedtime to allow your stomach to empty itself completely before your nightly fast.

Do this night limiter for two weeks straight before moving on.

TIME-RESTRICTED EATING (EIGHT TO NINE HOURS)

At this point, you've been at it for a month, practicing a twelve-hour fast and allowing the stomach to fully empty before bed. It is time to tighten up the eating window a squeak. Going forward, we are going to have a daily feeding window of eight to nine hours, rather than twelve hours. This will allow for a complimentary fifteen- to sixteen-hour fast.

Restricting your eating window to nine hours has been shown to have a significant benefit to your heart health. When we consider that cardiovascular disease is the number one killer of women in this country, followed closely by cancer, time-restricted eating is not only an awesome way to shed excess weight (and all the health conditions that come with being overweight), but it helps your quality of life and reduces your risk of major disease. Further evidence around stopping to eat at seven or eight o'clock in the evening is found in the literature around cancer and its recurrence.[115] While cancer is incredibly complicated, there is much speculation that it is a metabolic disease from lifestyle factors that can cause it as well. In fact, 65–75 percent of breast cancer risk is due to lifestyle!

Recent studies have shown fasting to have a huge benefit in the reduction of breast cancer risk, and reduction of recurrence if you've already had breast cancer.[116] For those of us who have already dealt with cancer, specifically breast cancer, research shows that practicing a daily fast will reduce the recurrence of breast cancer by 40 percent on its own, regardless of what your diet is. This means fasting alone decreases your risk for a relapse by 40 percent.

Isn't that incredible?

The bottom line here is we can grab hold of and control our lifestyle and reduce our risk and recurrence for breast cancers by 65–75 percent. More great news comes from research that shows profound effects on body weight in just twelve weeks of eight-hour time-restricted feeding.[117] These subjects limited food intake, eating between ten o'clock in the morning and six o'clock in the evening daily. They demonstrated decreases in body weight by ~3 percent relative to the control group. They also noted significant improvements in the reduction of systolic blood pressure relative to controls. The participants just ate what they normally ate, and researchers found the test subjects naturally consumed three hundred fewer calories per day. Some back of the envelope math says a reduction in three hundred calories daily over the course of a year equates to approximately thirty-one pounds of weight loss. This weight loss was achieved by simply restricting the eating window.

THE OMAD (AKA "TWENTY-FOUR HOUR FAST")

Once this eight to nine-hour fasting regimen is established and comfortable, we will begin to throw in a twenty-four-hour fast, once per week. You are still eating daily; you're just eating once per day. This might look like consuming breakfast one day and not eating until breakfast the following day or eating lunch and then abstaining from food until lunch the next day.

The first time you do this, you will feel hungry, especially around the time you usually eat. But don't panic, because hunger comes and goes in waves, and it shouldn't last longer than five to ten minutes. Water really helps to quell these hunger signals.

THE FREQUENCY OF YOUR FAST

The third lever to adjust is *how often* you engage in any one type of fast. Examples of changing your frequency can be daily, weekly, monthly, quarterly, or yearly. For example, I might engage in a *daily* time-restricted eating pattern, a *weekly* twenty-four-hour fast, a *monthly* seventy-two-hour fast, and a *yearly* five-day fast.

At the very minimum, I recommend practicing time-restricted eating daily, and depending on your hormonal status, you can play with some of the other levers of fasting to help amplify weight loss, energy, and breakthrough plateaus.

CYCLICAL FASTING: THROUGH YOUR CYCLE AND MENOPAUSE

After building up a tolerance to fasting by using the three levers (type, length, and frequency), we can now step it up and harmonize your fasting in a cyclical rhythm.

If you have a menstrual cycle and you are going to do a long fast that exceeds twenty-four hours, it is much better tolerated in the first two weeks of your cycle. If you recall from Chapter 3, estrogen and progesterone levels are relatively low at that time, and we are more receptive to the hormetic benefits of fasting. By contrast, the second half of our cycle, the luteal phase, is when we are generally the least receptive to long fasts, because our bodies are busy building up and using energy for thickening the endometrial lining.

For menopausal women, a fast can be done at any point in your four-week rotation, with longer fasts to be included when your carbohydrate intake is low. This would map out to week one and week three when you are following a 70 percent fat, 20 percent protein, 10 percent carbohydrate plan.

If you are shedding the old endometrial lining this week, your hormonal landscape is well suited for a fast that is multiple days in duration. If you are feeling up to it, this is the week to try a longer fast, and/or experiment with a caloric or non-caloric liquid fast. You might try a three-day caloric liquid fast this week with lots of bone broth to heal the gut. This fast is wonderful for a woman who knows she is estrogen dominant. Bone broth is rich in glycine, which activates growth hormone and helps with muscle repair. It is also involved in hemoglobin and myoglobin synthesis (which brings oxygen to muscle tissue), helps with engaging and maintaining sleep, and acts as an inhibitory neurotransmitter. It is also participating heavily in creatine synthesis, which is important when training anaerobically or with high intensity (like with heavy weights).

Depending on travel and stress levels, I will aim to fast for two to three days (forty-eight to seventy-two hours). I look at this as a time for "cleaning house."

An example fasting schedule this week might look like:

	Monday	Tuesday	Wednesday	Thursday	Friday	Saturday	Sunday
Fasting Type & Length	Time-Restricted Eating: 12 hours	Time-Restricted Eating: 12 hours	Time-Restricted Eating: 14 hours	Time-Restricted Eating: 16 hours	Caloric-Liquid Fast	Caloric Liquid Fast	Caloric Liquid Fast

As your womb is being cleaned out, it is a great opportunity to do the same with your digestive system. You should select the type of fast that best suits your hormonal profile (you can go back to Chapters 4 and 5 for a refresher). If you choose a non-caloric liquid fast, make sure green teas are part of your arsenal.

Green teas have a compound called EGCG, a potent sirtuin activator.[118] *Sirtuins* are involved in repairing DNA damage from the wear and tear of everyday life. In other words, sirtuin activation keeps us young! Over time, we learned sirtuins lose their ability to continue repairing at the speed they once did. Luckily, sirtuins are also activated when we are in a fasted state, when we are cold, or when we restrict macronutrients (like in a ketogenic diet). The more we can drive sirtuin activation, the younger we are on a cellular level.

Now we know that cold showers, the ketogenic diet, and fasting are ways for our sirtuins to continuously activate and repair damage. And as a vain woman who is driven to look and feel her best, what I can muster here is the more we can activate these sirtuins, the younger we can look and feel, and the longer we can live.

BEFORE OVULATION / WEEK TWO

For women with a cycle, your period is done, and you feel like the belle of the ball. Estrogen is rising to plump up your lips and cheeks (a sign of fertility), and testosterone is rising to make you feel like your sexy self.

Go you.

As with food, there are guidelines I like to honor in the fasting realms for women. I am a big proponent of building and maintaining lean muscle mass, so I don't recommend aggressive fasting this week. This week, we want to be driving muscle protein synthesis with both our exercises (these are outlined in Chapter 12) and our diet. I always joke after a heavy lift that I need to feed my legs, because they are hungry and need to repair!

I've also seen aggressive fasting affect ovulation, and just to err on the side of caution, I like only time-restricted feeding in week two. This recommendation applies for all hormonal types *except those with high testosterone.*

Ladies with PCOS or high testosterone can engage in several twenty-four-hour water fasts this week. The strategy behind this is to bring down insulin levels and therefore help luteinizing hormone (LH) surge to help release the egg.

For menopausal women, as you increase your protein this week to drive muscle protein synthesis, I typically recommend engaging only in time-restricted feeding this week. This can be a twelve-, fourteen- or sixteen-hour daily fast during this week.

An example fasting schedule for this week might look like this:

	Monday	Tuesday	Wednesday	Thursday	Friday	Saturday	Sunday
Fasting Type & Length	Time-Restricted Eating: 16 hours	Time-Restricted Eating: 16 hours	Time-Restricted Eating: 16 hours	Time-Restricted Eating: 16 hours	Time-Restricted Eating: 16 hours	Time-Restricted Eating: 16 hours	Time-Restricted Eating: 16 hours

AFTER OVULATION / WEEK THREE

In practice and in my personal life, I have seen a varying degree of success with long fasts (longer than twenty-four hours) in the last two weeks of a cycle, so the protocols we discuss will vary based on hormonal status, previous fasting experience, and tolerance.

As a general rule, it is harder to engage in a longer fast in your luteal phase. This is because there are a lot of metabolic changes

happening, like increasing glucose, fatty acids, and protein utilization. In other words, your body is using more calories to
drive the development of the endometrial lining.

There are usually two types of women I recommend continue
long-term fasting into the luteal phase of their cycle: women
with excess estrogen or testosterone.

Women with excess estrogen (estrogen dominance), will better
tolerate longer luteal fasts, as the digestive rest helps to reduce
inflammation, promote water excretion, and eliminate the water
weight and bloating often associated with excess estrogen and
PMDD. In fact, a bone broth fast for twenty-four hours sprinkled throughout weeks three and four will help improve gut
health and estrogen elimination.

For women with PCOS, there are often other issues like insulin
dysregulation, and fasting will help to sensitize your cells to
insulin. Women, as a whole, tend to be more insulin resistant
in the luteal phase of our cycles, and women with PCOS are
even more so. I have found this population responds well to
stricter forms of fasting in the luteal phase.

With this in mind, there is a ramping up in the luteal cycle in
terms of length and type of fast. Progesterone is beginning her
rise in week three, as well as her potent stimulation of your
appetite. She is also slowing down your bowel movements and
gobbling up serotonin to build out the endometrium.

For ladies with PMS, high estrogen, or low progesterone, we
want to ramp up liver detoxification, and promote bowel clearance to eliminate estrogen. Your fasting selection can include
one or more bone broth (caloric liquid) or water fasts.

For ladies with PCOS or high testosterone, I typically recommend water or herbal tea fasts. These can be sprinkled throughout the week or combined with a two- or three-day fast.

For my low testosterone and low estrogen ladies, aim for time-restricted eating of 16:8 this week.

Here's a sample fasting schedule for women with estrogen dominance:

	Monday	Tuesday	Wednesday	Thursday	Friday	Saturday	Sunday
Fasting Type & Length	Time-Restricted Eating: 16 hours	Caloric Liquid Fast	Time-Restricted Eating: 16 hours	Time-Restricted Eating: 16 hours	Caloric Liquid Fast	Time-Restricted Eating: 16 hours	Time-Restricted Eating: 16 hours

A sample fasting schedule for women with testosterone dominance:

	Monday	Tuesday	Wednesday	Thursday	Friday	Saturday	Sunday
Fasting Type & Length	Water-Only 24h Fast	Time-Restricted Eating: 16 hours	Water-Only 24h Fast	Time-Restricted Eating: 16 hours	Water-Only 24h Fast	Time-Restricted Eating: 16 hours	Time-Restricted Eating: 16 hours

A sample menopausal fasting rhythm:

	Monday	Tuesday	Wednesday	Thursday	Friday	Saturday	Sunday
Fasting Type & Length	Water-Only 24h Fast	Time-Restricted Eating: 16 hours	Time-Restricted Eating: 16 hours	Time-Restricted Eating: 16 hours	Time-Restricted Eating: 16 hours	Time-Restricted Eating: 16 hours	Time-Restricted Eating: 16 hours

BEFORE YOUR PERIOD / WEEK FOUR

Typically, this is the most difficult of all the weeks in your cycle to engage in fasting. As a whole, we are more insulin resistant in the luteal phase, with the apex of progesterone in Week Four potentially aggravating many chronic illnesses and disease states. Progesterone drives up serotonin usage, lipids, and proteins. We will see our appetite and cravings peak, our mood lower, and sleep disturbances increase. If you track your basal body temperature, you will notice a progressive increase in temperature this week.

With diet, it is often hardest to follow a lower carbohydrate or keto diet this week. As the endometrial lining thickenings, there is a continued increase in protein and fat requirements. Many of the symptoms associated with PMS affect blood sugar control. When estrogen levels are naturally high, your body may be resistant to its own insulin. For these reasons, irrespective of hormonal status, short stints of caloric liquid fasting for twenty-four hours or less are appropriate. The protein and other constituents found in bone broth can help thicken the lining of the endometrium. The protein will also help you feel full and can help with joint aches and pains.

In other words, ladies, let's just give ourselves a break this week and continue to practice time-restricting feeding without any long fasts. An example of fasting this week might look like:

	Monday	Tuesday	Wednesday	Thursday	Friday	Saturday	Sunday
Fasting Type & Length	Time-Restricted Eating: 14 hours	Time-Restricted Eating: 14 hours	Time-Restricted Eating: 14 hours	Time-Restricted Eating: 14 hours	Time-Restricted Eating: 14 hours	Time-Restricted Eating: 14 hours	Time-Restricted Eating: 14 hours

WHAT YOU CAN DO THIS WEEK

Work to build up your fasting tolerance slowly. Start with week one of the fasting tolerance protocol outlined in this chapter, and be gentle with yourself! Things like travel, poor sleep, stress at home and at work can all influence our ability to fast. Remember, the number one rule of a fast is to go slow and listen to your body!

You wouldn't yell at a baby for not knowing how to walk, right? You give her lots of tummy time, allow her to crawl, and support her as she learns to sit, then stand, and eventually walk. Give yourself the same grace and allow for this to be an opportunity for you to get to know yourself even better.

CHAPTER 11

ESSENTIAL SUPPLEMENTS

Imagine you are a huntress, living with your tribe ten thousand years ago. You have spent the day outdoors, tending to your garden planted in mineral-rich soil, and caring for the animals that roam freely. You have, along with the other women in your tribe, cleaned, fed, played with, and tended to the collective children. Your strong legs have taken somewhere around twenty-five thousand steps, lifting, squatting, bending, running, and walking with little or no footwear. Your hair is naturally highlighted from the sun, and your skin is golden. You sit under the stars, in the fresh air with your family, and eat dinner together. You retire to your quarters and moisturize your body with olive oil; you have pressed from your own olives. You have sex with your partner without time constraints or pressure. You go to sleep when it's dark and wake with the sun, perfectly attuned to the circadian rhythm of mother earth and the moon.

A divine existence, indeed. Now, contrast that with modern human life.

We spend the day indoors, under artificial lighting, bathing our biology in Wi-Fi. We grab highly processed, fast foods. We sit at a desk with little to no movement throughout the day. We hunch over our phones, constantly distracted by emails, social media, and devastating news. Our fitness devices whine and buzz that we haven't yet met our ten thousand steps today. We would probably only hit a few thousand steps if it weren't for the other indoor institution we frequent: the gym. We go there first thing in the morning, or at the end of the day, and we lift artificial weights eight to ten times or run endless miles on a cardio machine.

We get our pesticide-laden vegetables from the industrial agriculture complex that values quantity over quality. Soils are not rested or rotated to build up mineral content. Pesticides that are sprayed on crops run downstream, killing small field animals, and when they reach bodies of water, they kill our marine life. Animals are fed corn, sugar, and feces. (Yes, feces!) They live in crowded indoor quarters and generally live miserable lives until they are killed brutally and without mercy.

In grocery stores, food corporations use confusing terminology like "all-natural" and "fat-free" and use checkmarks from antiquated national institutions funded by profiteering pharmaceutical companies. We pick these franken-foods off the shelf thinking they are good for our bodies.

The deal is—even if you are eating a clean, whole food diet like The Estima Diet or Keto Cycling as we've outlined, chances are you are not getting all the nutrients you need because our soils are depleted, we unintentionally ingest herbicides, and we don't eat wild plants. This is why supplementation is important.

Some people initially resist supplements and say they prefer to get all their nutrients from their food. While it would be ideal to get all of our cellular requirements met from food, given the state of modern society, agriculture, and food mining practices, it is simply impossible. Supplements have gone from supplementing our diets to a necessary insurance policy to make sure we are properly nourished. Even with the best intentions, we still may not be getting the nutrients we need. We need to supplement to ensure we are getting the foundational basics into our bodies.

I have outlined the supplements I think every woman should take daily, along with dosages, time of day, and the point in your cycle where appropriate. These will help you combat common female mineral deficiencies, improve digestion, amp up liver detoxification, balance hormones, and improve glucose disposal.

FOUNDATIONAL SUPPLEMENTS
VITAMIN D3: SUNSHINE AND FAT LOSS IN A BOTTLE

Thanks to low-fat diets, sunscreen, and spending most of our time indoors, most people have suboptimal levels of vitamin D3.[119] Vitamin D3 is synthesized from cholesterol and is involved in almost every system in the body. In supplement form, it is a fat-soluble vitamin, meaning it can only be absorbed in the presence of fat. It helps shed belly fat, is intimately involved in bone density and helps with heart health.[120] In practice, I have most of my females take a minimum of 4000 IU/day throughout the year. In the summertime, as long as my patients pinky promise they will spend twenty to thirty minutes outdoors, we reduce it to 2000 IU/day. In the wintertime, with less sun exposure, and especially in women who are prone to seasonal affective disorder, my dosing recommendations climb to 6000 IU/day.

Pro tip: Take vitamin D3 with fat or with a meal. Or take it with some fat like olive oil straight up if you're a gangster.

Vitamin D3 supplementation shouldn't change throughout your cycle. It should remain at a consistent 2000 IU/day in the summer months, and up to 6000 IU/day in the winter months, or when you are not getting enough natural light.

MAGNESIUM: BETTER THAN DIAMONDS

Forget diamonds, Betty. Magnesium is a girl's best friend. Magnesium is the most abundant mineral in the body and the second most common dietary deficiency, second only to Vitamin D3. A deficiency in magnesium will raise blood sugar and insulin resistance (the exact opposite of what this book is trying to accomplish!), increase neural excitation, and contribute to our hedonic relationship with chocolate.[121] Part of the reason we crave chocolate around our period is because chocolate is an excellent source of magnesium.

Leafy green vegetables like the ones you will eat on The Estima Diet are a rich source of magnesium, and will, along with supplementation, work to correct any deficiency. If you suffer from PMS, magnesium is your girl.

Pro tip: Take magnesium in the evening, as it has sedative effects on blood sugar and calms the nervous system down.

A typical daily dose of magnesium is 200–400 mg. For the first two weeks of your cycle, aim to take 200–400 mg per day. In the second two weeks of your cycle, and especially if you suffer from PMS, I recommend a daily, divided dose of 800 mg. Meaning you will take 400 mg in the morning, and another 400 mg in the evening, with or without food.

OMEGA-3: SKIN, HAIR AND NAILS FOR DAYS

Our ancestors did not have to worry about refined sugars, grains, and vegetable oils. Today, these inflammatory foods make up over 70 percent of a typical western diet. And because we consume so much of these foods, they will, by default, replace minimally processed wild plant and animal foods, which will drive up inflammation.

This inflammation is represented by an increase in omega-6 fatty acids.[122] The ideal balance of omega-6s to omega-3s is 1:1. Some estimates have seen our modern lifestyle increase this ratio to as much as 20:1![123] This means that we, as a modern society, take in a huge amount omega-6 fatty acids relative to our omega-3s. Supplementing to balance this out is paramount.

There are two types of omega-3 fatty acids: eicosapentaenoic acid (EPA) and docosahexaenoic acid (DHA). These omega-3 fats are abundant in fish (hence the common term "fish oil"). Omega-3s are all about counteracting inflammation. And as we've discussed, you cannot lose weight if you are inflamed. Omega-3s have been shown to aggressively reduce triglyceride levels, and more modestly reduce blood pressure in hypertensives.[124] Being that cardiovascular disease is still the number one killer in women, heart health is of paramount importance, ladies.

I like to start most patients who are chronically stressed and complain of brain fog with a minimum of 3,000 mg to 3,500 mg of omega-3s, with a minimum of 1,000 mg coming from DHA. Once we bring down the inflammation, I reduce it to 2,000 mg on an ongoing basis. This does not change through the cycle and remains constant.

Pro tip: Take these supplements with a meal. So often, people will reject this supplement because of the "fish burp'" that may come when they are taken on an empty stomach. If you take them immediately before consuming a meal, the food is "on top" of the fish oil and won't give you that fishy aftertaste.

B12: ENERGY EXCELSIOR

B12 is a vitamin that is intimately connected with energy and methylation. Methylation is the process of adding a methyl group to a molecule. Even though this seems rather abstract, consider what methyl groups control:

- The stress (fight or flight) response
- The production and recycling of glutathione, the body's master antioxidant
- The detoxification of hormones, chemicals, and heavy metals
- The inflammation response
- Genetic expression and the repair of DNA
- Neurotransmitters and the balancing of brain chemistry
- Energy production
- The repair of cells damaged by free radicals
- The immune response, controlling T-cell production, fighting infections and viruses, and regulating the immune response

Given that these are pretty important functions, it is important to make sure our B12 levels are in check. B12 also plays a vital role in brain health, heart health, and our immune system.[125]

A daily dose of 1,000 mcg (1 mg) is sufficient as a daily dose throughout your cycle with no need for modification from the follicular to luteal phase.

BERBERINE: LET THEM EAT CAKE

Berberine has been used in Chinese and Ayurvedic medicine for centuries. Berberine is an excellent way to reduce insulin resistance, fasting glucose, and blood sugar levels.[126] There is robust evidence that suggests taking 1,500 mg of berberine in three divided daily doses is equivalent to taking popular medications used to treat Type 2 Diabetes. Berberine has also been shown to aid in weight loss, boost metabolism, reduce inflammation, help with liver and gut health, and boost memory.[127]

For my women with excess estrogen or excess testosterone, this supplement is the belle of the ball; taking it before a meal will help lower blood glucose. So, if you happen to be at a party or family gathering and your favorite cake is there, have this on hand in your clutch and take it right before you eat a slice.

COLLAGEN: SMOOTH AS A BABY'S BOTTOM

As we age, our collagen levels naturally begin to decline. Because collagen is the most abundant protein in the body, this decline will affect every part that has connective tissue, including our muscles, hair, bones, joints, discs, heart, liver, and even our blood cells!

Unfortunately, where we first begin to see signs of collagen degradation is in our skin and muscles—they begin to lose their firmness and sag over time.[128] I consume hydrolyzed collagen daily, a specific type of collagen that is easy to absorb because the amino acids in the collagen are already assembled and ready for use. Hydrolyzed collagen gives your body small useable chunks of peptides that are easily absorbed and used by the body. I will have this either in my coffee or in a post-workout recovery shake.

Like berberine, there are stacks and stacks of evidence supporting hydrolyzed collagen as a means to improve skin hydration, elasticity, and firmness, as well as positively impacting bone density.[129] If you're a vain woman like me, then collagen will become one of the prized supplements in your Betty arsenal.

CURCUMIN: INFLAMMATION BE GONE!

Curcumin is the active ingredient in turmeric, and if you love Indian food as I do, you are well acquainted with its distinctive yellow pigment in curry. It is a powerful antioxidant and almost magical at bringing down all markers of inflammation in the body. It helps the body produce more of its own antioxidants,[130] and several studies have demonstrated its ability to improve the symptoms of depression, joint pain, and osteoarthritis.[131]

If you are chronically stressed, a minimum of 3 g/day in divided doses works well. Depending on the severity of inflammation, supplementation of up to 8 g is considered safe with no side effects.

HORMONAL CUSTOMIZATION

The supplements discussed in this chapter are foundational

basics. Meaning every woman, irrespective of menstrual or hormonal status, should be taking these stacks as a way to optimize her biology. There are also add-on supplements you can pair with the hormones we outlined in Chapters 2, 3, 4, and 5. I have also included additional supplementation protocols with dosages and timing to consider in the charts below. You may need some of them, or all of them. And remember, you cannot supplement your way out of a bad diet! Like their name suggests, they are *supplements* to the classic Estima Protocol, Period Cycling, and Fasting Protocols in Chapters 8, 9, and 10. If you are on a budget, start with the foundational basics described in this chapter, and slowly add these in over time, as needed.

The Estima Method Protocol—Chronic Inflammation, High Cortisol and Stress

- Berberine: 1,500 mg/day in three divided doses
- Hydrolyzed Collagen: one scoop/day
- Curcumin: 3 g/day in three divided doses
- Magnesium: 400 mg/day, in the evening
- Omega-3s: 3,000–3,500 mg/day in divided doses
- Vitamin C: 3,000 mg/day in three divided doses
- Vitamin D: 4,000 IU/day

The Estima Method Protocol—High Estrogen or Low Progesterone

- Berberine: 1,500 mg/day in three divided doses
- Broccoli Seed Extract: 100 mg/day
- Curcumin: 3 g/day in three divided doses
- Diindolylmethane (DIM): 100 mg/day, can double to 200 mg/day in luteal cycle
- Green Tea Extract: 100 mg/day

- Hydrolyzed Collagen: one scoop/day
- Magnesium: 400 mg/day, in the evening
- Omega-3s: 3,000–3,500 mg/day in divided doses
- Vitex Agnus-Castus: 200 mg/day

The Estima Method Protocol—High Testosterone

- Berberine: 1,500 mg/day in three divided doses
- Broccoli Seed Extract: 100 mg/day
- Curcumin: 3 g/day in three divided doses
- Hydrolyzed Collagen: one scoop/day
- Magnesium: 400 mg/day, in the evening
- Omega-3s: 3,000–3,500 mg/day in divided doses
- Zinc: 30 mg/day

The Estima Method Protocol—Low Testosterone

- Curcumin: 3 g/day in three divided doses
- DHEA: 10 mg/day in divided doses
- Horny Goat Weed: 250 mg in divided doses
- Hydrolyzed Collagen: one scoop/day
- Magnesium: 400 mg/day, in the evening
- Omega-3s: 3,000–3,500 mg/day in divided doses

The Estima Method Protocol—Low Estrogen

- Black Cohosh: 20–40 mg/day
- Curcumin: 3 g/day in three divided doses
- DHEA: 10 mg/day
- Gingko Extract: 100 mg/day in divided doses
- Hydrolyzed Collagen: one scoop/day
- Maca: 1,500–3,000 mg/day
- Magnesium: 400 mg/day, in the evening

- Omega-3s: 3,000–3,500 mg/day in divided doses
- Panax Ginseng: 100 mg/day in two divided doses

WHAT YOU CAN DO THIS WEEK

Start with the recommended foundational supplements outlined in this chapter. I recommend trying the foundational basics for a few months first. This gets you in the habit of taking your supplements daily and is enough of a runway to begin noticing differences in yourself.

CHAPTER 12

GO TO THE GYM, SHE SAID. IT'LL BE FUN, SHE SAID.

I have a drug for you.

This drug will allow you to have more energy, sleep at night, reduce your anxiety, make you horny, sharpen your thinking, keep you feeling young, and is as effective (if not more) than any anti-depressant you've ever taken.[132]

This drug is exercise.

I should mention, as a considerable bonus, this drug has no side effects, and you can refill the prescription as often as you want. And best of all? It's *free*. And unlike most other drugs that are touted to be a cure-all miracle, this drug truly is the one that delivers on that lofty promise. Exercise is the key to youthful energy, better sex, a better mood, and a long life. And yet, when I speak with women who are not regularly exercising, I often hear things like their schedules are too busy for exercise, they're too tired at the beginning or end of the day, or they don't know where to start.

While it may be true that I could have written another book about exercise entirely, this chapter will start your roadmap to getting fit, building muscle, and feeling strong again. I am reticent to say anything is proven in science. Science isn't something that "settles," but exercise is the exception to this rule. Exercise, beyond a shadow of a doubt, is proven to be good for your health. Think of any parameter that might define good health such as cardiovascular conditioning, brain health, mental health, menstrual pain, stress reduction, or hormonal balancing. Exercise positively benefits them all. You name it, and study after study has shown the beneficial effects of exercise.[133]

I pinky promise you that this drug, exercise, will work for you. But, like any other drug, in order for it to exert its effects, you have to take it.

STRONG LIKE A BULL AND LIVING PAST ONE HUNDRED

I have this vision of when I am one hundred years old. I am still able to lift the equivalent of a suitcase into the overhead compartment of a plane (because, obviously, I am traveling back and forth between my villa in the Bordeaux region of France and wherever my sons live). I can pick up my great-grandchildren, get down on the floor and play with them, and still have the strategic brain to beat my grandchildren in a game of Italian cards. But in order for me to do these things, I need to lift weights.

Developing muscle right now and continuing to do so as we age is important because muscle mass directly correlates with our metabolism.[134] Muscle is functional, active tissue, meaning the maintenance of our active tissue will require the expenditure of more calories. In other words, more muscle naturally burns more calories to maintain itself. More muscle is also synonymous with better glucose control, because our muscles act like a glucose sink—they sop up all the excess in and out of the bloodstream.

Outside the liver, the muscles are the largest reservoir of glycogen (which is stored as glucose) in the body. And unlike the liver, once glucose gets into the muscles, it cannot get out. The glucose becomes trapped inside the muscle for use exclusively by the muscle. Sort of like Vegas, right? When glucose gets into your muscles, it *stays* in your muscles. And remember, bones and muscles are twins. When we have more muscle mass, our bones are denser, and the opposite is also true: when we have less muscle, our bones degenerate and become weak and frail.

And just like with our diet, there are important considerations for an exercise program to be effective for women. The first problem is that we generally don't move as much throughout the day as we probably ought to. This general movement is referred to as NEAT (non-exercise activity thermogenesis). This is the low-level daily activity our foremothers engaged in while they were harvesting food from the land, tending to the children, and cooking. Low-level activity all throughout the day meant they were movement *generalists*. Contrast this activity to that of the modern-day woman, who is more of a movement *specialist*, meaning she likely attends a class or goes to the gym for a specific workout and then sits for the rest of the day. Engaging in general movement contributes to your caloric expenditure and consists of non-specific movements. Examples of NEAT-inspired movements are going for a walk, gardening, and cleaning the house like your mother-in-law is coming over. Or maybe that last one is just me? I clean the floors like I mean it before my in-laws come over!

Another major issue I see in most female exercise plans is we do not train in all the ways our body was designed to move, in many planes of movement. So much of our movement is restricted to one type of motion, like flexion and extension of our limbs, while keeping them close to the midline. This is movement along the *sagittal plane*. Just take a look at your typical cardio machines at the gym for an example. Most of them keep your arms and legs close to the midline, while moving your legs forward and backward. The treadmill has you flexing and extending the hips and knees, while keeping your arms near your waist, flexing and extending the shoulder and the elbow. Same goes for the elliptical machine, the stair climber, and the bike—they all have identical movement patterns built into them.

I am not saying these movements are bad; it is the fact that these movements make up the commanding majority in our exercise programs that I take issue with. The issue I have with *only* engaging in this type of movement is that it reinforces the movement we do all day anyway: flexion. We *already* sit flexed over a desk, slouched in the car, and neck-craning forward over our phones all day, with our arms by our sides. We *already* play in the sagittal plane in everyday life as it is. By only engaging in flexion and extension movements with our limbs hanging out in the midline, we lose out on the opportunity to work and train our lateral muscles (like our shoulders, glutes, and much of our abdominals) as these muscles either start or end by attaching to bones on the lateral parts of the body. And when we are building out a well-rounded training program, it should take into account a variety of movements.

THE CORONAL PLANE

For women, let's begin to consider more movements where you move your arms and legs away from the midline, in the coronal plane. This plane of movement is all about moving out to the side, away from, or crossing the midline. Some examples of coronal plane movements might be jumping jacks (arms and legs go out the side and then return), curtsy squats (squats with one leg crossing behind the other), side to side lunges, skater squats, and warrior two pose in yoga.

These exercises are highly specific to developing the muscles on the side of the body—the glutes, the shoulders, and the oblique muscles, to name a few. This is incredibly important for women because our hips, which are anatomically wider than men's, are designed to shake, sway, and move in a figure-eight pattern. Developing our glutes not only make us look amazing in a pair of jeans, but they provide stability to the hips and keep our bones strong as we age. Remember, muscles and bones are twin sisters. When one is strong, so is the other. Weak, atrophied muscle can and will contribute to decreasing bone density over time.

LOOK MA, NO HANDS!

For women, the ability to get up out of a chair unassisted or get up off the floor using no arms is one of the biggest predictors of longevity.[135] Yes, that means getting up without using your hands. To be able to do this requires relying solely on the strength of your glutes, core, and the proprioceptive feedback from the associated joints in your hips, knees, ankles, and spine.

If your muscles are weak, then your bones will be frail, accelerating joint destruction and making fractures, slips, and falls a likely possibility as you age. If you are unfortunate enough to know a woman who has fractured her hip, you will likely have also observed her cognitive capacity decline alone with it. Hip fractures are associated with six times more cognitive decline in women in the following years versus their peers without fractures.[136] In other words, if you fracture your hip with an unintended fall, your mobility, flexibility, strength, and brain health will all suffer as a result. We want to prevent this now by developing as much strength through our pelvis as possible.

And while I admittedly love to train my legs, upper body strength is an incredibly important consideration for women, as we are notoriously weaker than men in the upper extremity. So much so that we even have pushups that are "modified" for us and called a "women's pushup." I'm sorry Betty, but no. We should be able to punch out pushups on our toes and have the strength to lift things without straining or throwing our backs out. Think of push-ups as squats for the upper body. You should be training regularly for progress!

No matter where you are in your exercise journey, we are going to dive into how we can play around with movement therapy, including rehabilitation and resistance training to build strength, more muscle, and keep you feeling like a million bucks. Remember, practice makes progress, and that is what we are going for!

DEFINE YOUR GOALS AND DREAMS

Whether you are a beginner or an advanced exerciser, there are a few key things we want to establish before designing any type of exercise routine. First, and most importantly—what are your goals and dreams for your body?

I can chirp all day long about the importance of muscles, but what is it that *you* want? Why is building muscle, or even contemplating more exercise important *to you*? Let's ponder a few questions and write the answers down.

When you think about your body, how do you want to feel living in it?

If you were to achieve the goals you have for your body, describe an average day for you and how it would feel.

WHAT ARE SOME OF THE AREAS OF YOUR BODY YOU WOULD LIKE TO BE STRONGER?

Is flexibility a goal for you? What about explosive power? Speed? Balance? Describe how these will benefit you in your life.

How do you feel about your posture?

Do you have any aches and pains in your body that need to be attended to?

What feels right about your body right now? Name the things you love about your body and why you love them.

Defining your desires for your body, both in terms of aesthetics and function, will help you focus on the next action steps you can take for yourself. It is perfectly alright to have aesthetic goals as long as you practice love and compassion for the body you have *right now*, with the sole intention of tweaking and improving upon the masterpiece you already own. Remember, you can be healthy, beautiful, and sexy simply by deciding you are, not only when you attain a goal in the future. You are all of those things right now if you decide them to be true.

If you're having trouble embracing the idea that you're already a gorgeous drop-dead sexy bombshell, start with appreciating your body. How your body has dutifully served you with unrestricted breath and oxygenated blood. She has maintained a heartbeat and a pulse, has delivered oxygen to your cells, maintained a certain posture, and metabolized countless meals without you ever having to think about or consciously direct those actions. Can you imagine how exhausting it would be to tell your heart to beat sixty times every minute, while remembering to also take in fifteen breaths every minute, *and* tell your cells that they need to make more energy? Your body is a wonderland of geeky magic, and it's important to recognize this right now and always. Start from a place of love and gratitude for all that your body has done, its wildly magical capabilities, and know that, you, the eternal student, can improve how you function, look, and feel.

If you have identified that you have some rehabilitation, aches and pains, or a history of previous injures, I highly recommend seeking out a chiropractor or bodyworker you know and trust to help you work through these issues manually. In the following sections, we will outline movements and rehabilitation exercises, and how to grow some beautiful, strong muscles.

ESTROGEN SAYS MIND YOUR TENDONS AND LIGAMENTS

Ever notice sometimes when you do yoga or other basic stretches you are stiff as anything, and other times, you can practically put your feet behind your head? This is not an accident. If you are still in your reproductive years, your tendons and ligaments will change over the course of the month, so there will be times when your ligaments are looser (we call this laxity), and times when your tendons will stiffen up. This is because our tendons and ligaments are highly influenced by the ever-changing peaks and valleys of estrogen during our cycle.[137]

In other words, when estrogen is high, our ligaments get looser, and our tendons get stiffer. If you start paying attention, you might notice how "flexible" you are right around ovulation but much less during your period. Ligaments like the ACL ligament in the knee show a direct relationship between laxity and rupture,[138] meaning the laxer it is, the greater chance it can be injured, with the potential to rupture. Not surprisingly, women in their reproductive years have far more ACL injuries than their male counterparts, and this is directly attributable to our peaks and valleys of estrogen during our cycle.

If you recall from Chapter 3, the second week of your cycle is where we see the highest rise in estrogen, just ahead of ovulation. Estrogen peaks in week two to drive the maturation of the follicle and the egg, but in doing so, she makes our ligaments lax and our tendons stiff. Consequently, at this time in our cycle, we should reduce explosive power movements that impart a lot of force upon the ligaments. I typically discourage plyometric exercises like burpees, jumping squats, or sprinting in week two because that's when our ligaments are much more susceptible to injury.

Estrogen levels also influence the *type* of injuries women sustain, which is distinct from our male counterparts. Women in their reproductive years tend to suffer fewer muscle injuries, but more ligament injuries than men, and this is because of the increased ligamentous laxity we experience throughout the month. This changes when we are menopausal. We will tend to get fewer ligament injuries but will be more susceptible to muscle injuries.

Now our tendons, unlike our ligaments, become stiffer under estrogen's influence. And stiff tendons are wonderful for lifting weights. This is because tendons are able to maintain joint stability and prevent injuries under tension. A tendon with proper stiffness will transfer force from muscle to bone and create the movement. And with an increase in estrogen right before we ovulate, this means our tendons will be stiffer, which is great for lifting heavy weights.

This is also why it is so important to heal any estrogen dominant hormonal issues. Recall from Chapter 4 that estrogen dominance begins in our mid-thirties as progesterone begins to decline. If the tendon is too stiff (because of too much estrogen) it will not stretch, and then the muscle you are trying to contract is forced to lengthen. This is bad news bears for my estrogen-dominant Bettys, because now the muscle attached to this super stiff tendon will experience more lengthening for any movement, including contraction. This is where we can injure our muscles and tendons.

As a general rule, when developing an exercise program that has explosive movements like plyometrics, take a few days off on either side of ovulation and opt for heavy weights instead. If you are tracking your cycle, I'd cut the plyometrics from about day eleven of your cycle to day fifteen. Instead, as you will see, when we design your weight training program, you can use this time to lift heavy weights, as your tendons are best suited for bigger weights during this time. You can resume plyometrics in the other weeks of your cycle, being mindful that your estrogen is lowest in your bleed week and in the days leading up to your period. That means these times are ideal for burpees, jumping onto park benches, and sprinting.

BUILDING BEAUTIFUL MUSCLES

Lifting weights is the easiest way to reshape your body, improve body composition, and recalibrate your metabolism. And it is no surprise that as our menstrual cycle dictates the nutrient composition and calories we take in; it also influences our training schedule.

Designing an exercise regimen is highly specific to the individual, but as a general rule of thumb, you need to perform around ten sets of any given exercise per week to grow that muscle.[139] So, if you are looking to build a round booty, there needs to be a minimum of ten booty-building sets per week. Let's say squats are going to be a part of your booty building arsenal. You might split your training over three days, meaning that on Monday, you might do three sets of squats (you'll see how many reps to do based on your cycle in the next section), three sets of squats on Wednesday, and four sets on Friday. This will give you the ten-set minimum to begin lifting, sculpting, and rounding out your glutes.

And before you even have time to think it, let me tell you that even though you are engaging in muscle hypertrophy by adhering to this ten-set rule, by no means will you turn into the Hulk. Pinky swear, Betty. You simply do not have enough testosterone to drive that kind of growth. The misinformation around women and muscle building is astonishing and still persists today.

Now, the great thing about growing muscles is it is more important to work the muscle to fatigue than it is to adhere to a certain number of repetitions. Meaning that eight reps of a moderate weight that bring the muscle to exhaustion will have a similar effect as twenty reps at a lighter weight. The only thing that has to happen consistently is the muscle needs to be worked to fatigue. A clue to what works for you is the last three reps should be challenging, maybe even necessitating a spotter or someone to help you polish off the set.

When we take the basic principles of muscle growth (ten sets per week and the muscle must be fatigued in each set) and couple it with hormonal variance and our changing ligaments and tendons, this offers us the opportunity to modify our workouts throughout the month while continuing to make gains. I typically like to choose between five and six exercises for every workout, but I may do more or less depending on the quality of my sleep, if I'm travelling, or how much energy I have.

If you are new to weight training, starting with two to three days of training per week is usually appropriate. You might consider one full-body, one upper-body, and one lower-body workout. If you have more experience with weights, consider designing a four- or five-day split with specific focus on certain body parts for each one. When I do this, I will typically choose a "push" and a "pull" movement. For example, day one might be biceps (pull) with triceps (push), day two might be glutes (push),and hamstrings (pull), day three might be chest (push) and back (pull), and day four might be another round of legs. I have included a sample of what each breakdown might look like below.

SAMPLE BEGINNER WEIGHT TRAINING WORKOUT—THREE DAYS A WEEK

Monday: Full Body (four sets, circuit format*)

Reverse Lunge to Curtsy Lunge

Push-ups

Sumo Squat

One arm dumbbell row

Plank with Alternating Knee to Shoulder

Glute Bridge with Abduction at Top

*Circuit means you do all the exercises listed in a row, and once you finish, begin at the first exercise again

Wednesday: Upper Body and Abs with Giant* Sets

Criss-Cross Cycling Abs	Giant Set: five sets of each
Assisted Pull Ups	
Reverse Flys	
Plank with Alternating Knee to Shoulder	Giant Set: five sets of each
Push-ups – four count down, four count up	
Dumbbell Overhead Press	
Plank In and Out	Giant Set: five sets of each
Plank: Alternating Elbows to Hands	
Dumbbell Lateral Deltoid Raise	

*Giant sets are three different exercise performed in a row

Friday: Lower Body Giant Sets

Curtsy Squat with Abduction	Giant Set: four sets of each
Reverse Frog Lifts	
Weighted Glute Bridges with Pulse at Top	

Sumo Squat	Giant Set: four sets of each
Reverse Lunge	
Deadlifts	

Banded Giant Walks	Giant Set: four sets of each
Squat With three Abductions at Bottom	
Hamstring Curls with Exercise Ball	

If you want to see me sweat through this workout you can head over to www.bettybodybook.com/bonus for the video and instructions.

SAMPLE INTERMEDIATE WEIGHT TRAINING—FOUR DAY SPLIT

If you are a more seasoned weightlifting queen, you might consider a four-day split where you divide body parts more deliberately. Consider the following example of a four-day split I have used:

Monday: Arms and Abs

Lumber Jack Abs Crunch	Three sets of each
Tricep Dips with Weighted Vest	
Bicep Curl – Supine Grip	

Hanging Ab Crunches	Giant Set: five sets of each
Skull Crusher Tricep Extension	
Push-ups	

Plank In and Out	Giant Set: five sets of each
Tricep Push-up	
Bicep Curl – Prone Grip	

Tuesday: Legs

Hip Thrust with Weight	Three sets of each
Banded Jumping Squats	
Banded Giant Walk	

Hamstring Curl with Exercise Ball	Giant Set: five sets of each
Sumo 1.5 Squats	
Deadlifts	

Banded Curtsy Squat with Abduction	Giant Set: five sets of each
Banded Reverse Frog Lifts	
Alternating Reverse Lunges	

Wednesday: Rest

Thursday: Upper Body

Band Assisted Chin-Ups	Three sets of each
Seated Incline Chest Press	
Lateral Deltoid Raise	

Barbell Bent Over Row	Giant Set: five sets of each
Seated Overhead Shoulder Press	
Spiderman Push-ups on Bench	

Seated Lateral Row	Giant Set: five sets of each
Reverse Flys	
Dumbbell Front Raise	

Friday: Legs

Hip Thrust with Weight	Three sets of each
Banded Jumping Squats	
Banded Giant Walk	
Ass to the Grass Squat	Four sets
Reverse Lunge to Curtsy Lunge	Four sets
One legged Banded Hip Thrust	Four sets
Deadlift	Four sets
Kettlebell Swings	Four sets
Assisted One Legged Pistol Squat	Four sets

For videos on these exercises, head over to www.bettybodybook.com/bonus.

EXERCISE CYCLING

With the above templates, you can see that a well-rounded training program includes many angles and planes of movement for best results. You may have noticed that the templates omit repetitions within each set. This is because I like to run these templates through a cyclical filter, as we have been doing through much of this book. When you are in your reproductive years, you can use these templates for altering repetitions to coincide with the hormonal environment you are housing that week.

BLEED WEEK / WEEK ONE

When beginning your period, the first day or so might leave you feeling tired and sluggish. Be gentle with yourself here and remember you are shedding an organ. If you are feeling achy or tired, give yourself a break, Betty. Instead of weights on the first day or so of your period, opt for yoga or lower intensity activities like walking or light stretching. As you get into the rhythm of your period, transition to moderate weights, meaning your repetitions might fall into the ten to fifteen repetition range, with the last three repetitions being difficult to complete.

You may consider adding in some high-intensity interval training this week as well. You can add a quick ten-minute set at the end of your weight training or do it as a separate workout. Recall that estrogen is low this week, making your ligaments less lax and well suited for explosive power.

WEEK BEFORE OVULATION / WEEK TWO

As you are coming off your period and moving towards ovulation, your testosterone is reaching its highest peak in your cycle this week. If you recall from Chapter 3, this peak in testosterone will help you feel flirty, sexy, and horny. This week is the perfect time to use heavy weights to compliment testosterone's peak and drive up your capacity to create muscle mass. In other words—go heavy with the weights! You will also have more natural energy, so use it to your advantage.

A good rule of thumb for lifting heavy weights is to aim for five to seven reps, where your muscles are close to failure by the fifth repetition. I always recommend a spotter when possible when you are first starting out. Aiming for ten sets to drive muscle growth, I will often do four to five sets of any given exercise because the repetitions are shorter (5–7).

As estrogen peaks this week to drive follicular maturation, I'd back off the explosive power cardio moves this week, as this is where we see more ligamentous laxity and an overall female-specific decrease in power output. Steady-state cardio is the cardio of choice this week. I typically dance to my favorite songs, use a rebounder (a mini-trampoline), or go for long bike rides or runs alternate to my heavy lift days.

AFTER OVULATION / WEEK THREE

After ovulation, as our energy moves inward, I like to back off the heavy weights and transition into the moderate weights described in the bleed week. For resistance training, that means completing ten to fifteen repetitions of moderate weight.

Estrogen declines rapidly immediately after ovulation, and then just as suddenly, begins a secondary rise of the month. This week is a great time to drive stimuli to connective tissue and enhance balance and proprioception. Alternating resistance training days with yoga days are a great way to honor and protect your tendons, ligaments, and muscles. Better cardio choices include steady-state activities that eliminate burst or explosion movements, since they don't place much strain on ligaments.

BEFORE YOUR PERIOD / WEEK FOUR

The week right before your period is a week to back off on heavy weights and engage in higher repetitions, aiming for between fifteen to twenty repetitions of any given exercise. I have found that mentally, women tend to feel better with lighter weights and higher repetitions. You can explore what feels best for you, keeping in mind that the muscle should be worked to fatigue. Estrogen and progesterone decline midweek, making this another wonderful time for high-intensity interval training, although you may not necessarily be in the mood for it!

Being more inflamed is normal right before your period. If

your hormones are dysregulated and imbalanced, this week can be particularly difficult. Remember to listen to your body and give her what she needs. Sleep disturbances this week can affect our mood and desire to lift heavy, so I love to lighten the weight and go for higher repetitions—usually between fifteen and twenty per exercise.

And think about it: you've spent the last three weeks lifting moderate and heavy weights. It is time to let yourself recover, repair, and gain strength so you can continue to make gains. Pushing yourself and ignoring the value of recovery this week is a recipe for injury and regression. Remember, recovery is where all your gains come from. If you do not take the time to recover, your body will hold on to fat like an insurance policy because you are overdriving stress signals. Give yourself permission to rest. It took me a while to accept this week in particular, but once I did, I made much faster gains in my physique, my strength, and my power.

You may find that continuing high repetitions of fifteen to twenty reps for the first few days of your period can be helpful to continue training while being easier on your body. This is especially true if you find yourself to be sluggish the first few days.

DEVELOPING GREAT POSTURE

Posture rehabilitation is another important consideration when remodeling the look and function of your body. Many women want long, graceful necks and to permanently relieve the ongoing tension residing in our neck and shoulders. Modern-day living necessitates our shoulders to hike up, with waning mobility and flexibility. Let's do a quick check-in, Betty: does the rotation of the head from side to side seem more difficult these days? What about bringing your ear down to your shoulder? What about tipping your head back?

With hours spent logged into our computers and phones, a lack of generalized movement during the day like walking, or even failing to change your position at your desk frequently, we develop poor posture. This is because we are changing the way our joints move in relation to one another, and the length of our tendons and ligaments change. Muscular asymmetry develops, and some become short and tight while others become long and weakened.

Experience tells me that it is much easier for you to flex your head forward and bring your chin to your chest than it is for you to extend your neck backwards, mouth closed without discomfort or hearing creaks and cricks in your neck. I would also guess that if you were to start from a neutral position and rotate your head to look toward your shoulder, it would be difficult for you to line up your nose and shoulder without extending your head backward or rotating your shoulder forward. These two motions, extension and rotation, are the first two we begin to lose as we age because we barely do them. It is as simple as use it or lose it.

Now, I am the first to say there is no one "perfect" posture. Posture, in an ideal world, would be an ever-changing one because we'd dynamically change our body position with lots of general movement. But the reality is, we barely move. We might, if we are lucky, get one workout in at the beginning or end of the day and spend the remainder of the day sitting at desks and in meetings. Those sedentary hours are spent with our head tipped slightly forward, with the muscles in the front of our neck getting short and tight and the muscles on the back of our neck getting long and weak.

And of course, as we mentioned in Chapter 6, if we're in this flexed position all the time, our muscles will start to assume these positions even when we are not doing them. If you recall from Chapter 6, this is called *physiological creep*. And as muscles and bones are twins, this creep will begin to destroy the natural curves in our neck and our low back.

The curve in our neck, known as lordosis, is designed to load the weight of the head, as well as protect the spinal cord that lives inside it. Your head weighs about the same as a bowling ball, somewhere between twelve and fifteen pounds. If you imagine holding a bowling ball, the easiest way to do so is to bend your elbow and keep it close to your body, so you could exert the least amount of effort to hold it. But what if you extended your arm, still holding the bowling ball? Over time, it would be much harder, wouldn't it? This is because you increase what is known as the *moment arm* or lever arm. If the heaviest part of your upper body, your head, is always forward, the joints in your neck feel like they're holding a bowling ball with an extended arm. This wears out the muscles, and they will eventually fail.

The problem is, with so many things to focus on in everyday life, finding yet another window of time for posture rehabilitation is another item on the to-do list that will likely never happen. Ben Greenfield, author of *Boundless*, first introduced me to the concept of "movement snacks," which I thought was brilliant. The idea is that we take five- or ten-minute movement breaks through the day to walk, do rehab exercises, or stretch. Basically, you take the time to do what you know you *should* be doing.

Think about it, if you take six little movement snacks, each lasting about ten minutes, you've magically found an entire hour every day to work on your posture and get your rehab in. The possibility for movement snacks is endless! You could go for a walk, or even get in some big multi-joint exercises like squats or lunges in between video calls and meetings. It also breaks up the monotony of computer work, and keeps your brain oxygenated and sharp.

With all this to consider, the best place to start to reverse poor posture is to retrain and strengthen the muscles that extend and rotate and improve flexibility in the muscles that flex the neck and the low back. No matter how much damage your neck or low back has endured, the great news is that it can always be improved. Our skeleton completely remodels itself every two to three years, and with the right input, like the exercises outlined below, you can improve not only the quality of your bones, but the curves of your spine, and the balance and symmetry of your muscles.

For a full list of posture rehabilitation exercises, head over to www.bettybodybook.com/bonus.

Here are a few of my favorite rehabilitation exercises to integrate into your workday or after a workout:

STARGAZER STRETCH

This is a glorious stretch for the sternocleidomastoid muscle, which is the muscle that helps with neck flexion and rotation. This muscle gets notoriously tight in people who work over laptops. This stretch can be done several times a day, holding for thirty seconds each side.

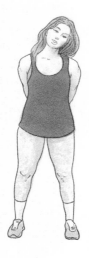 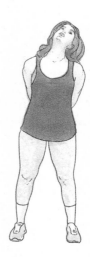

FOLLOW THE FINGER

This is a great exercise for incorporating both extension and rotation in your neck, two movements we do not get enough of in daily life. I like to do this at my desk, doing one side ten times, and repeating on the other side. You can set a timer on your phone and do this every hour on the hour all day, and it feels phenomenal.

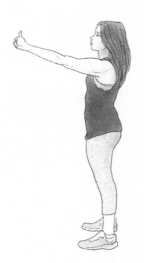 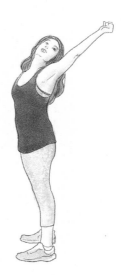

CHICKEN CHINS

This exercise addresses the long and weak muscles in the back of the neck. Notice how my chin is elevated and not in neutral. Neutral chin tucks do nothing for the curve in your neck, and I'd argue they work to flatten the curve rather than promote it. With the chin elevated, we are helping to restore the natural lordotic curve of the neck.

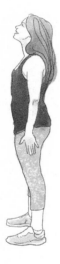 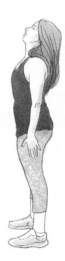

MULTIFIDUS STABILITY

One of the consequences of sitting all day is atrophy of our multifidus muscle—one of the major contributors to proprioception and stability in the spine. This exercise works on the opposite side of the arm that is moving.

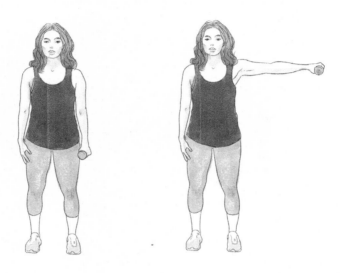

SIDE TO SIDE ABS

When crunches get boring, try these fun twists to engage your core. I do these while I'm brushing my teeth in the morning!

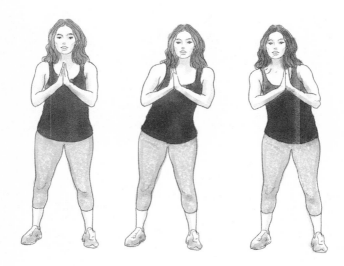

These postural exercises will compound in their effect over time. They are designed to improve your active range of motion, retrain and reset overly tense muscles, and build your flexibility. Not only is this important for relieving the common tension in our spines, but it will allow for better ligament and tendon health and prevent injuries that can occur from imbalances.

THINGS YOU CAN DO THIS WEEK

Think about the goals you have for yourself and why you want them. Is it a longevity play? To look great on your upcoming vacation? To help amplify the effects of the diet? All of the above? Thinking and journaling about what you want from your exercise journey will help you stick with it when you feel like quitting.

CHAPTER 13

BETTY—IS THAT YOU?

Squeak! You've finished reading the book. Ah. Ma. Gad. What a feat and an accomplishment! You are one of the special ones who made a commitment and followed through to the end. You are one of us now, Betty. A hardcore truth seeker who knows that aging isn't where your posture melts down like a taper candle. You know you can have limitless energy, reset your metabolism, be strong at any age, and live in cyclical harmony on repeat, forever.

We've covered so much data, science, and protocols in this book, it can seem overwhelming and leave you in a tizzy as to where to begin. You have already unlocked a secret level by finishing this book. That was step one. Go, you! Already winning. Ah, I pick my Bettys so good.

The next step is the transcendence of information into application. Applying what you have read in a reasonable, measurable way gets you winning. It is like the old adage says, "How do you eat an elephant? One bite at a time." So, your very next bite is to decide which pieces of this book are you going to apply. Go back through the chapters and select ten things you want to introduce or accomplish in your life, in no particular order.

BUILDING OUT YOUR BETTY BLUEPRINT

Now that you have ten, we are going to pick one (yes, just one) thing for you to master in the next few weeks. Are you taking the orgasm challenge? Aiming to get eight hours of sleep? Building up your fasting tolerance? It truly doesn't matter which one it is. The point is I want to help you overcome the inertia of inaction and just *start*. Pick the topic you want to focus on and commit to it. You might go through the book in chronological order how it's laid out, or you may prefer skipping to specific topics you want to focus on, like the Estima Diet or building an evening routine. Just pick one thing and pinky promise yourself that you will do your very best to work on it for the next four weeks. This isn't about being perfect, it is about progress and moving your needle on that subject a little closer to mastery. Repeat this month-long process with each of the ten items you have chosen and promise yourself you will ease into the processes of this book like a gorgeous dress. Let the changes take on your shape, as you are ready for them to do so. Give yourself a month to really master each chapter, and rinse and repeat as often as needed.

This is the beginning of a roadmap, a ten-month runway to give yourself the grace, permission, and ease to peel back the petals and reveal more of you. And truthfully, working one-on-one with patients in the clinic, it takes about nine or ten months to start seeing real, lasting results from their efforts.

The next tool you need in your arsenal is a new mindset—a commitment to yourself, and knowing you are worth investing at least ten months in. None of us get through life unscathed, and all of us have baggage, trauma, and residue from our pasts. If the thought of releasing the things that you carry as a burden seems too big of an ask, I understand. What I will ask you to do is *temporarily suspend the disbelief* that you are anything less than a geeky magic wonderland. I promise you can go back to self-deprecating thoughts and sabotaging behaviors in due time, but only after you have given yourself this ten-month grace period.

You may find that after learning to love yourself, nourishing the temple that is your body, and attuning to your natural cyclical rhythms, you quite like how it makes you feel. Dare I suggest maybe keep some of it for the long ride, too? Maybe. Possibly. Just a squeak.

This is a healing mindset embodied. Carol Dweck, author of the seminal book, *Mindset*, describes the difference between a growth mindset and a fixed mindset. You have the tools laid out in this book, and now your mind needs to help with the execution. In other words, you need to believe you are worth investing in. A fixed mindset focuses on whether you fail, how many times you fail, and trying to live up to an impossible measure of what success looks like. Someone with a fixed mindset has a hard time believing that things could ever be marginally different than the way they are right now.

On the contrary, someone like you has the beginnings of a growth mindset. You are open and ready for change, you understand that your thoughts become reality, and whether you think you can, or you cannot, you are right. After all, here you are at the end of this book! Don't focus too much on the gap between where you are now and where you want to be. Know that it is constantly changing and every day you commit to this protocol, you are closing the gap.

So, how do you know if you're making progress? Do you

remember how you felt ten months ago? Yeah, me neither. The answer to this puzzle is data collection. Start a journal, take your measurements, record your weight, and do the quizzes in the appendix section. Revisit these measurements, quantifiers, and qualifiers monthly. How can you look forward if you don't know where you stand right now? You can measure with an app, a bound journal by your bedstand, or your phone's memo recorder. I usually have a wearable fitness tracker that tells me how many steps I take, what my heart rate and sleep look like, and how many calories I burned that day. The app that accompanies these wearables can also act as your journal.

BE THE BABY GIRAFFE

Wherever you are in your journey, know this truth: change is hard but not impossible. Your body wants, *nay*, demands through her symptoms to pay attention to her! She has, in all her glory, the capacity for abundant health. As humans, we generally have disdain for being a beginner. We want to excel, and we want to excel right now. But I encourage you to think of a newborn baby giraffe when it is first born, with legs that are impossibly long, bendy, and all over the place. They wibble, wobble, and knock their knees multiple times before learning to stand. But all the bumps and bruises are worth it in the end. It is hard work, but after all the falls, retries, and fails, baby giraffe figures out how not to wrap her legs around her body.

Such is the paradox in life: the things worth having always take work. Be the baby giraffe. Be willing to fail, and even fall off track completely! Be willing to be a beginner and know at times it will be uncomfortable. Failing is a necessary part of being successful, Betty. You need to also know what does *not* work in order to move toward what does work. Continue to be willing to learn and persevere through the discomfort. Stand up for your body, your brain, and for the wondrous amalgamation of stardust that you are.

MY WISH FOR YOU

My wish for you is that you take pause and wonder at how glorious your body is. All the places she has taken you, leading you right up to this moment. Your body is alive, right here, right now. Right at this very moment she is working tirelessly for you: your heart lovingly pumping out blood and maintaining a certain blood pressure, your digestive system quietly absorbing nutrients from your last meal, and your billions of cells humming and producing energy as you need them to. In your falling in love with your physiology, I hope you will gain an appreciation for the only place you will ever live, and the only wealth you truly have—your body and your health. Your body is your temple and it is a wonder to be worshipped. I hope you realize you have everything inside of you to create the life you want. Here is your Wizard of Oz moment: everything you need is already inside of you, and you can come home to health whenever you want. You just need a few tools to help you get there, all of which have been outlined in this book. It is in settling into this awakening that you will discover yourself.

And hey, you do not need to do this alone. There are a bunch of Bettys waiting to meet you in our online community, and we would love to get to know you better! Every month we have live connection calls, new recipes, new workouts, new rehab exercises, new hormone balancing protocols, mindset, self-love, and actionable items to help you continue your Betty journey. We talk about sex (I mean, of course, we do), the divine masculine, the divine feminine, and how to love yourself like you mean it. We are the girlfriends and community you've always wanted and have been waiting for. Head over to www.hellobetty. club and check us out.

My vision for you is that you will begin to feel like your sparkly self again with the abundant energy and mental clarity you want. I want you to feel good in your skin, not because of a ruthless, punitive diet, but because you love yourself and celebrate your body. I want you to look at yourself and say, "Damn, girl, I am loving getting to know you!"

When I was in school, these principles of health were not taught. Women were "smaller men," or just smaller versions of men with pesky hormones. I had years where I rallied against my own menstrual cycle (and clearly lost). When I had my first great period, I had this inkling of a feeling—an intuitive knowing that it could be like this every month. I believed menstruation didn't have to be a harrowing, cramp-inducing foggy haze of tears and pain. I could fall in love with my period, and I could help other women who were willing to play and experiment and be my test subjects while I developed these protocols. We all know that you cannot medicate a problem you behaved your way into. But you can behave your way out of it.

You have read through all the science, complex physiological pathways, random brain facts, nutrition and exercise physiology, and of course, sex. You have in your hands my proven methods that I use with my private clients, and most of all, an understanding of *why*. You don't need to be a soldier just following orders. You have the "why" piece of the puzzle, so you can be the general of your own army. You are part of the Betty army now. You are home.

APPENDIX

COHEN PERCEIVED STRESS

The following questions ask about your feelings and thoughts during THE PAST MONTH.

In each question, you will be asked HOW OFTEN you felt or thought a certain way. Although some of the questions are similar, there are small differences between them, and you should treat each one as a separate question. The best approach is to answer fairly quickly. That is, don't try to count up the exact number of times you felt a particular way, but tell me the answer that in general seems the best.

For each statement, please tell me if you have had these thoughts or feelings: never, almost never, sometimes, fairly often, or very often (read all answer choices each time).

	Never	Almost Never	Sometimes	Fairly Often	Very Often
B1. In the past month, how often have you been upset because of something that happened unexpectedly?	0	1	2	3	4
B2. In the past month, how often have you felt unable to control the important things in your life?	0	1	2	3	4
B.3. In the past month, how often have you felt nervous or stressed?	0	1	2	3	4
B.4. In the past month, how often have you felt confident about your ability to handle personal problems?	0	1	2	3	4
B.5. In the past month, how often have you felt that things were going your way?	0	1	2	3	4
B.6. In the past month, how often have you found that you could not cope with all the things you had to do?	0	1	2	3	4
B.7. In the past month, how often have you been able to control irritations in your life?	0	1	2	3	4
B.8. In the past month, how often have you felt that you were on top of things?	0	1	2	3	4
B.9. In the past month, how often have you been angry because of things that happened that were outside of your control?	0	1	2	3	4
B.10. In the past month, how often have you felt that difficulties were piling up so high that you could not overcome them?	0	1	2	3	4

PERCEIVED STRESS SCALE SCORING

Each item is rated on a five-point scale ranging from never (o) to almost always (4). Positively worded items are reverse scored, and the ratings are summed, with higher scores indicating more perceived stress.

PSS-10 scores are obtained by reversing the scores on the four positive items: For example, 0=4, 1=3, 2=2, etc. and then summing across all ten items. Items 4, 5, 7, and 8 are the positively stated items.

Your Perceived Stress Level was _____

Scores around thirteen are considered average. In our own research, we have found that high-stress groups usually have a stress score of around twenty points. Scores of twenty or higher are considered high stress, and if you are in this range, you might consider learning new stress reduction techniques as well as increasing your exercise to at least three times a week. High psychological stress is associated with high blood pressure, higher BMI, larger waist to hip ratio, shorter telomere length, higher cortisol levels, suppressed immune function, decreased sleep, and increased alcohol consumption. These are all important risk factors for cardiovascular disease.

WEIGHT AND MEASUREMENTS SHEET

Throughout the program, weigh yourself daily to be sure you stay on track. Once a week, take your waist and hip measurements, and record both those and your weight on the sheet below.

Starting Measurement Date: _____

Starting Weight _____ lbs.

Starting Waist Measurement_____inches

Starting Hip Measurement _____inches

Measurement Date: _____

Weight _____ lbs.

Waist Measurement _____inches

Hip Measurement_____inches

Measurement Date: _____

Weight _____ lbs.

Waist Measurement _____inches

Hip Measurement_____inches

Measurement Date: _____

Weight _____ lbs.

Waist Measurement _____inches

Hip Measurement_____inches

Measurement Date: _____

Weight _____ lbs.

Waist Measurement _____inches

Hip Measurement_____inches

Measurement Date: _____

Weight _____ lbs.

Waist Measurement _____inches

Hip Measurement_____inches

ABOUT THE AUTHOR

DR. STEPHANIE is widely recognized as an expert in brain optimization, body composition, and metabolism with a specific application to female physiology.

She studied neuroscience and psychology and received her Bachelor of Science with Honors from the University of Toronto. She went on to complete her Doctor of Chiropractic degree at the Canadian Memorial Chiropractic College in 2003.

For more than fifteen years, she has worked with actors, professional athletes, entrepreneurs, and political leaders. She is an international speaker, and has been a top writer on Medium. com, Thrive Global of *The Huffington Post*, and a guest on numerous TV shows. She is the host of the acclaimed *Better! with Dr. Stephanie* podcast. Her online courses have reached thousands of women worldwide to reclaim and empower them to make better health decisions. She is a former figure competitor, placing third in the New York Regional Division, National Physique Committee.

Dr. Stephanie has an innate love for language, culture, and

cuisine and is particularly enamored with French, Italian, and Greek.

She has lived in Montreal, New York, London, and currently lives in Toronto with her husband and three children.

NOTES

1   "betty," Urban Dictionary, last modified June 23, 2013, https://www.urbandictionary.com/define.php?term=betty.

2   Adele Kennedy et al., "The Metabolic Significance of Leptin in Humans: Gender-Based Differences in Relationship to Adiposity, Insulin Sensitivity, and Energy Expenditure," *The Journal of Clinical Endocrinology & Metabolism* 82, no. 4 (April 1, 1997): 1293–1300, https://doi.org/10.1210/jcem.82.4.3859.

3   Women spend 50 percent more time doing unpaid work than men. Source: "Daily Average Time Spent in Hours on Various Activities by Age Group and Sex, 15 Years and Over, Canada and Provinces," Statistics Canada, last modified November 13, 2020, https://www150.statcan.gc.ca/t1/tbl1/en/tv.action?pid=4510001401.

4   "Women Shoulder the Responsibility of 'Unpaid Work'," Office for National Statistics, last modified November 10, 2016, https://www.ons.gov.uk/employmentandlabourmarket/peopleinwork/earningsandworkinghours/articles/womenshouldertheresponsibilityofunpaidwork/2016-11-10.

5   Elizabeth McCauley, "Americans Think Sex Should Determine Chores for Straight Couples, Masculinity and Femininity For Same-Sex Couples," American Sociological Association, https://www.asanet.org/sites/default/files/pr_am_2016_quadlin_news_release_final.pdf.

6   Mark P. Mattson, Valter D. Longo, and Michelle Harvie, "Impact of Intermittent Fasting on Health and Disease Processes," *Ageing Research Reviews* 39 (October 2017): 46–58, https://doi.org/10.1016/j.arr.2016.10.005.

    Mohammad Bagherniya et al., "The Effect of Fasting or Calorie Restriction on Autophagy Induction: A Review of the Literature," *Ageing Research Reviews* 47 (November 2018): 183–97, https://doi.org/10.1016/j.arr.2018.08.004.

Damien Roussel, Mélanie Boël, and Caroline Romestaing, "Fasting Enhances Mitochondrial Efficiency in Duckling Skeletal Muscle by Acting on the Substrate Oxidation System," *The Journal of Experimental Biology* 221, no. 4 (December 21, 2017), https://doi.org/10.1242/jeb.172213.

Cesare Granata, Nicholas A. Jamnick, and David J. Bishop, "Training-Induced Changes in Mitochondrial Content and Respiratory Function in Human Skeletal Muscle," *Sports Medicine* 48, no. 8 (June 22, 2018): 1809–28, https://doi.org/10.1007/s40279-018-0936-y.

Keliane Liberman et al., "The Effects of Exercise on Muscle Strength, Body Composition, Physical Functioning and the Inflammatory Profile of Older Adults," *Current Opinion in Clinical Nutrition & Metabolic Care* 20, no. 1 (January 2017): 30–53, https://doi.org/10.1097/mco.0000000000000335.

7   Shilpa Prasad et al., "Impact of Stress on Oocyte Quality and Reproductive Outcome," *Journal of Biomedical Science* 23, no. 1 (March 29, 2016), https://doi.org/10.1186/s12929-016-0253-4.

8   Ariana D. Majer et al., "Is There an Oxidative Cost of Acute Stress? Characterization, Implication of Glucocorticoids and Modulation by Prior Stress Experience," *Proceedings of the Royal Society B: Biological Sciences* 286, no. 1915 (November 13, 2019), https://doi.org/10.1098/rspb.2019.1698.

9   Vibha Rani et al., "Oxidative Stress and Metabolic Disorders: Pathogenesis and Therapeutic Strategies," *Life Sciences* 148 (March 2016): 183–93, https://doi.org/10.1016/j.lfs.2016.02.002.

10 "Biobehavioral Responses to Stress in Females: Tend-and-Befriend, Not Fight-or-Flight," in *Foundations in Social Neuroscience* (Cambridge, MA: The MIT Press, 2002), https://doi.org/10.7551/mitpress/3077.003.0048.

11 Christopher A. Brown, Christopher Cardoso, and Mark A. Ellenbogen, "A Meta-Analytic Review of the Correlation between Peripheral Oxytocin and Cortisol Concentrations," *Frontiers in Neuroendocrinology* 43 (October 2016): 19–27, https://doi.org/10.1016/j.yfrne.2016.11.001.

12 Kaori Watanabe and Taku Shirakawa, "Characteristics of Perceived Stress and Salivary Levels of Secretory Immunoglobulin A and Cortisol in Japanese Women With Premenstrual Syndrome," *Nursing and Midwifery Studies* 4, no. 2 (June 27, 2015), https://doi.org/10.17795/nmsjournal24795.

Nancy Fugate Woods, Ada Most, and Gretchen D. Longnecker, "Major Life Events, Daily Stressors, and Perimenstrual Symptoms," *Nursing Research* 34, no. 5 (September 1985): 263–267, https://doi.org/10.1097/00006199-198509000-00002.

Pauline M. Maki et al., "Menstrual Cycle Effects on Cortisol Responsivity and Emotional Retrieval Following a Psychosocial Stressor," *Hormones and Behavior* 74 (August 2015): 201–8, https://doi.org/10.1016/j.yhbeh.2015.06.023.

13 Maren Wolfram, Silja Bellingrath, and Brigitte M. Kudielka, "The Cortisol Awakening Response (CAR) across the Female Menstrual Cycle," *Psychoneuroendocrinology* 36, no. 6 (July 2011): 905–12, https://doi.org/10.1016/j.psyneuen.2010.12.006.

14   "Menstruation in Girls and Adolescents: Using the Menstrual Cycle as a Vital Sign,"
      Pediatrics 137, no. 3 (February 22, 2016), https://doi.org/10.1542/peds.2015-4480.

15   Tim Christen et al., "Sex Differences in Body Fat Distribution Are Related to Sex
      Differences in Serum Leptin and Adiponectin," *Peptides* 107 (September 2018): 25–31,
      https://doi.org/10.1016/j.peptides.2018.07.008.

16   Johannes Fuss et al., "Masturbation to Orgasm Stimulates the Release of the
      Endocannabinoid 2-Arachidonoylglycerol in Humans," *The Journal of Sexual Medicine* 14,
      no. 11 (November 2017): 1372–79, https://doi.org/10.1016/j.jsxm.2017.09.016.

17   M. Mihm, S. Gangooly, and S. Muttukrishna, "The Normal Menstrual Cycle in Women,"
      Animal Reproduction Science 124, no. 3–4 (April 2011): 229–36, https://doi.org/10.1016/j.
      anireprosci.2010.08.030.

      Robert L Barbieri, "The Endocrinology of the Menstrual Cycle," in *Methods
      in Molecular Biology*, 145–69 (New York: Springer New York, 2014), https://doi.
      org/10.1007/978-1-4939-0659-8_7.

18   S.G. Hillier, "Current Concepts of the Roles of Follicle Stimulating Hormone and
      Luteinizing Hormone in Folliculogenesis," *Human Reproduction* 9, no. 2 (February 1994):
      188–91, https://doi.org/10.1093/oxfordjournals.humrep.a138480.

19   Clarisa R. Gracia et al., "Predictors of Decreased Libido in Women during the Late
      Reproductive Years," *Menopause* 25, no. 11 (November 2018): 1238–43, https://doi.
      org/10.1097/gme.0000000000001225.

20   Oleg Varlamov, Cynthia L. Bethea, and Charles T. Roberts, "Sex-Specific Differences in
      Lipid and Glucose Metabolism," *Frontiers in Endocrinology* 5 (January 19, 2015), https://doi.
      org/10.3389/fendo.2014.00241.

      M. Wallace et al., "Effects of Menstrual Cycle Phase on Metabolomic Profiles in
      Premenopausal Women," *Human Reproduction* 25, no. 4 (February 10, 2010): 949–56,
      https://doi.org/10.1093/humrep/deq011.

      C. F. Draper et al., "Menstrual Cycle Rhythmicity: Metabolic Patterns in Healthy Women,"
      Scientific Reports 8, no. 1 (October 1, 2018), https://doi.org/10.1038/s41598-018-32647-0.

21   A. K. Fong, and M. J. Kretsch, "Changes in Dietary Intake, Urinary Nitrogen, and Urinary
      Volume across the Menstrual Cycle," *The American Journal of Clinical Nutrition* 57, no. 1
      (January 1, 1993): 43–46, https://doi.org/10.1093/ajcn/57.1.43.

22   Junaidah B. Barnett et al., "Plasma Lipid and Lipoprotein Levels during the Follicular and
      Luteal Phases of the Menstrual Cycle," *The Journal of Clinical Endocrinology & Metabolism*
      89, no. 2 (February 2004): 776–82, https://doi.org/10.1210/jc.2003-030506.

23   Jennifer M. Rutkowsky et al., "Acylcarnitines Activate Proinflammatory Signaling
      Pathways," *American Journal of Physiology-Endocrinology and Metabolism* 306, no. 12 (June
      15, 2014): 1378–87, https://doi.org/10.1152/ajpendo.00656.2013.

24 Manuel Mai et al., "Serum Levels of Acylcarnitines Are Altered in Prediabetic Conditions," ed. Bin He, *PLoS ONE* 8, no. 12 (December 16, 2013), https://doi.org/10.1371/journal.pone.0082459.

25 Alexandros Tsoupras, Ronan Lordan, and Ioannis Zabetakis, "Inflammation, Not Cholesterol, Is a Cause of Chronic Disease," *Nutrients* 10, no. 5 (May 12, 2018): 604, https://doi.org/10.3390/nu10050604.

26 Ilaria Paterni, Carlotta Granchi, and Filippo Minutolo, "Risks and Benefits Related to Alimentary Exposure to Xenoestrogens," *Critical Reviews in Food Science and Nutrition* 57, no. 16 (May 25, 2017): 3384–3404, https://doi.org/10.1080/10408398.2015.1126547.

27 Dimitrios Agas, Giovanna Lacava, and Maria Giovanna Sabbieti, "Bone and Bone Marrow Disruption by Endocrine-Active Substances," *Journal of Cellular Physiology* 234, no. 1 (June 28, 2018): 192–213, https://doi.org/10.1002/jcp.26837.

Dimitrios Agas, Maria Giovanna Sabbieti, and Luigi Marchetti, "Endocrine Disruptors and Bone Metabolism," *Archives of Toxicology* 87, no. 4 (November 29, 2012): 735–51, https://doi.org/10.1007/s00204-012-0988-y.

S.V. Fernandez and J. Russo, "Estrogen and Xenoestrogens in Breast Cancer," *Toxicologic Pathology* 38, no. 1 (November 21, 2009): 110–22, https://doi.org/10.1177/0192623309354108.

28 Kok-Yong Chin, Kok-Lun Pang, and Wun Fui Mark-Lee, "A Review on the Effects of Bisphenol A and Its Derivatives on Skeletal Health," *International Journal of Medical Sciences* 15, no. 10 (2018): 1043–50, https://doi.org/10.7150/ijms.25634.

29 Victoria Lloyd et al., "Hormone-Like Effects of Bisphenol A on P53 and Estrogen Receptor Alpha in Breast Cancer Cells," *BioResearch Open Access* 8, no. 1 (October 1, 2019): 169–84, https://doi.org/10.1089/biores.2018.0048.

30 Ying Liu, Nhi Nguyen, and Graham A Colditz, "Links between Alcohol Consumption and Breast Cancer: A Look at the Evidence," *Women's Health* 11, no. 1 (January 2015): 65–77, https://doi.org/10.2217/whe.14.62.

31 Siriporn Thongprakaisang et al., "Glyphosate Induces Human Breast Cancer Cells Growth via Estrogen Receptors," *Food and Chemical Toxicology* 59 (September 2013): 129–36, https://doi.org/10.1016/j.fct.2013.05.057.

32 Elaine Stur et al., "Glyphosate-Based Herbicides at Low Doses Affect Canonical Pathways in Estrogen Positive and Negative Breast Cancer Cell Lines," ed. Aamir Ahmad, *PLOS ONE* 14, no. 7 (July 11, 2019), https://doi.org/10.1371/journal.pone.0219610.

33 Dagfinn Aune et al., "Fruit and Vegetable Intake and the Risk of Cardiovascular Disease, Total Cancer and All-Cause Mortality—a Systematic Review and Dose-Response Meta-Analysis of Prospective Studies," *International Journal of Epidemiology* 46, no. 3 (February 22, 2017): 1029–56, https://doi.org/10.1093/ije/dyw319.

X. Wang et al., "Fruit and Vegetable Consumption and Mortality from All Causes, Cardiovascular Disease, and Cancer: Systematic Review and Dose-Response Meta-Analysis of Prospective Cohort Studies," *BMJ* 349, no. 3 (July 29, 2014): 4490–4490. https://doi.org/10.1136/bmj.g4490.

J. Kapusta-Duch et al., "The Beneficial Effects of Brassica Vegetables on Human Health," *Roczniki Panstwowego Zakladu Higieny* 63, no. 4 (2012): 389–95, http://citeseerx.ist.psu. edu/viewdoc/download?doi=10.1.1.871.8734&rep=rep1&type=pdf.

Dorette T.H. Verhoeven et al., "A Review of Mechanisms Underlying Anticarcinogenicity by Brassica Vegetables," *Chemico-Biological Interactions* 103, no. 2 (February 1997): 79–129, https://doi.org/10.1016/s0009-2797(96)03745-3.

Yang Bai et al., "Sulforaphane Protects against Cardiovascular Disease via Nrf2 Activation," *Oxidative Medicine and Cellular Longevity* (2015): 1–13, https://doi.org/10.1155/2015/407580.

Joseph P. Burnett et al., "Sulforaphane Enhances the Anticancer Activity of Taxanes against Triple Negative Breast Cancer by Killing Cancer Stem Cells," *Cancer Letters* 394 (May 2017): 52–64, https://doi.org/10.1016/j.canlet.2017.02.023.

34 Ju-Hee Lee et al., "Sulforaphane Induced Adipolysis via Hormone Sensitive Lipase Activation, Regulated by AMPK Signaling Pathway," *Biochemical and Biophysical Research Communications* 426, no. 4 (October 2012): 492–97, https://doi.org/10.1016/j. bbrc.2012.08.107.

Marcos Roberto de Oliveira, Flávia di Bittencourt Brasil, and Cristina Ribas Fürstenau, "Sulforaphane Promotes Mitochondrial Protection in SH-SY5Y Cells Exposed to Hydrogen Peroxide by an Nrf2-Dependent Mechanism," *Molecular Neurobiology* 55, no. 6 (July 20, 2017): 4777–87, https://doi.org/10.1007/s12035-017-0684-2.

35 Anastasiya Slyepchenko et al., "Intestinal Dysbiosis, Gut Hyperpermeability and Bacterial Translocation: Missing Links Between Depression, Obesity and Type 2 Diabetes," *Current Pharmaceutical Design* 22, no. 40 (December 14, 2016): 6087–6106, https://doi.org/10.2174/ 1381612822666160922165706.

Tao Yang et al., "Gut Dysbiosis Is Linked to Hypertension," *Hypertension* 65, no. 6 (June 2015): 1331–40, https://doi.org/10.1161/hypertensionaha.115.05315.

Lisa Rizzetto et al., "Connecting the Immune System, Systemic Chronic Inflammation and the Gut Microbiome: The Role of Sex," *Journal of Autoimmunity* 92 (August 2018): 12–34, https://doi.org/10.1016/j.jaut.2018.05.008.

Marta Anna Szychlinska et al., "A Correlation between Intestinal Microbiota Dysbiosis and Osteoarthritis," *Heliyon* 5, no. 1 (January 2019), https://doi.org/10.1016/j.heliyon.2019. e01134.

36 Zeina Haoula et al., "Lipidomic Analysis of Plasma Samples from Women with Polycystic Ovary Syndrome," *Metabolomics* 11, no. 3 (August 17, 2014): 657–66, https://doi. org/10.1007/s11306-014-0726-y.

Paolo Moghetti, "Insulin Resistance and Polycystic Ovary Syndrome," *Current Pharmaceutical Design* 22, no. 36 (November 11, 2016): 5526–34, https://doi.org/10.2174/1381 612822666160720155855.

Seema Patel, "Polycystic Ovary Syndrome (PCOS), an Inflammatory, Systemic, Lifestyle Endocrinopathy," *The Journal of Steroid Biochemistry and Molecular Biology* 182 (September 2018): 27–36, https://doi.org/10.1016/j.jsbmb.2018.04.008.

37   Sarah Kent and Richard Legro, "Polycystic Ovary Syndrome in Adolescents," Adolescent
     Medicine 13, no. 1 (March 2002): 73–88.

38   Stefano Palomba et al., "Pregnancy Complications in Women with Polycystic Ovary
     Syndrome," Human Reproduction Update 21, no. 5 (June 27, 2015): 575–92, https://doi.
     org/10.1093/humupd/dmv029.

39   Neil F. Goodman et al., "American Association of Clinical Endocrinologists, American
     College of Endocrinology, and Androgen Excess and PCOS Society Disease State Clinical
     Review: Guide to the Best Practices in the Evaluation and Treatment of Polycystic Ovary
     Syndrome—Part 1," Endocrine Practice 21, no. 11 (November 2015): 1291–1300, https://doi.
     org/10.4158/ep15748.dsc.

40   Birinder S. Cheema, Lisa Vizza, and Soji Swaraj, "Progressive Resistance Training in
     Polycystic Ovary Syndrome: Can Pumping Iron Improve Clinical Outcomes?" Sports
     Medicine 44, no. 9 (May 29, 2014): 1197–1207, https://doi.org/10.1007/s40279-014-0206-6.

     Antonio Paoli et al., "Effects of a Ketogenic Diet in Overweight Women with Polycystic
     Ovary Syndrome," Journal of Translational Medicine 18, no. 1 (February 27, 2020), https://
     doi.org/10.1186/s12967-020-02277-0.

41   Jakob L. Vingren et al., "Testosterone Physiology in Resistance Exercise and
     Training," Sports Medicine 40, no. 12 (December 2010): 1037–53, https://doi.
     org/10.2165/11536910-000000000-00000.

42   N. Geary, "The Effect of Estrogen on Appetite," Medscape Womens Health 3, no. 6
     (November 1998): 3.

43   Michael J. Keenan et al., "Role of Resistant Starch in Improving Gut Health, Adiposity,
     and Insulin Resistance," Advances in Nutrition 6, no. 2 (March 1, 2015): 198–205, https://doi.
     org/10.3945/an.114.007419.

     Laure B. Bindels et al., "Resistant Starch Can Improve Insulin Sensitivity Independently
     of the Gut Microbiota," Microbiome 5, no. 1 (February 7, 2017), https://doi.org/10.1186/
     s40168-017-0230-5.

     Christopher L et al., "Resistant Starch and Protein Intake Enhances Fat Oxidation and
     Feelings of Fullness in Lean and Overweight/Obese Women," Nutrition Journal 14, no. 1
     (October 29, 2015), https://doi.org/10.1186/s12937-015-0104-2.

44   Julian Meyer Berger, et al., "Mediation of the Acute Stress Response by the Skeleton," Cell
     Metabolism 30, no. 5 (November 2019): 890-902, https://doi.org/10.1016/j.cmet.2019.08.012.

45   Wenyu Huang et al., "Circadian Rhythms, Sleep, and Metabolism," Journal of Clinical
     Investigation 121, no. 6 (June 1, 2011): 2133–41, https://doi.org/10.1172/jci46043.

46   Michael R. Irwin, Richard Olmstead, and Judith E. Carroll, "Sleep Disturbance, Sleep
     Duration, and Inflammation: A Systematic Review and Meta-Analysis of Cohort Studies
     and Experimental Sleep Deprivation," Biological Psychiatry 80, no. 1 (July 2016): 40–52,
     https://doi.org/10.1016/j.biopsych.2015.05.014.

47 Kenneth Lo et al., "Subjective Sleep Quality, Blood Pressure, and Hypertension: A Meta-Analysis," *The Journal of Clinical Hypertension* 20, no. 3 (February 19, 2018): 592–605, https://doi.org/10.1111/jch.13220.

Li Chengyang et al., "Short-Term Memory Deficits Correlate with Hippocampal-Thalamic Functional Connectivity Alterations Following Acute Sleep Restriction," *Brain Imaging and Behavior* 11, no. 4 (July 21, 2016): 954–63, https://doi.org/10.1007/s11682-016-9570-1.

48 Rachel P. Ogilvie and Sanjay R. Patel, "The Epidemiology of Sleep and Obesity," *Sleep Health* 3, no. 5 (October 2017): 383–88, https://doi.org/10.1016/j.sleh.2017.07.013.

Long Zhai, Hua Zhang, and Dongfeng Zhang, "Sleep Duration and Depression Among Adults: A Meta-Analysis of Prospective Studies," *Depression and Anxiety* 32, no. 9 (June 5, 2015): 664–70, https://doi.org/10.1002/da.22386.

Min Young Chun et al., "Association between Sleep Duration and Musculoskeletal Pain," *Medicine* 97, no. 50 (December 2018), https://doi.org/10.1097/md.0000000000013656.

Sohrab Amiri, and Sepideh Behnezhad, "Sleep Disturbances and Back Pain," *Neuropsychiatrie* 34, no. 2 (March 12, 2020): 74–84, https://doi.org/10.1007/s40211-020-00339-9.

49 Sirimon Reutrakul, and Eve Van Cauter, "Sleep Influences on Obesity, Insulin Resistance, and Risk of Type 2 Diabetes," *Metabolism* 84 (July 2018): 56–66, https://doi.org/10.1016/j.metabol.2018.02.010.

Tianyi Huang et al., "Habitual Sleep Quality and Diurnal Rhythms of Salivary Cortisol and Dehydroepiandrosterone in Postmenopausal Women," *Psychoneuroendocrinology* 84 (October 2017): 172–80, https://doi.org/10.1016/j.psyneuen.2017.07.484.

William D.S. Killgore, "Effects of Sleep Deprivation on Cognition," in *Progress in Brain Research* (New York: Elsevier, 2010), 105–29, https://doi.org/10.1016/b978-0-444-53702-7.00007-5.

50 "Sleep and Sleep Disorder Statistics," American Sleep Association, last modified November 15, 2020, http://www.sleepassociation.org/about-sleep/sleep-statistics.

51 Monica L. Andersen et al., "The Association of Testosterone, Sleep, and Sexual Function in Men and Women," *Brain Research* 1416 (October 2011): 80–104, https://doi.org/10.1016/j.brainres.2011.07.060.

52 David A. Kalmbach et al., "The Impact of Sleep on Female Sexual Response and Behavior: A Pilot Study," *The Journal of Sexual Medicine* 12, no. 5 (May 2015): 1221–32, https://doi.org/10.1111/jsm.12858.

53 Parisa Vidafar et al., "Increased Vulnerability to Attentional Failure during Acute Sleep Deprivation in Women Depends on Menstrual Phase," *Sleep* 41, no. 8 (May 22, 2018), https://doi.org/10.1093/sleep/zsy098.

54 H. S. Driver, "Sleep and the Sleep Electroencephalogram across the Menstrual Cycle in Young Healthy Women," *Journal of Clinical Endocrinology & Metabolism* 81, no. 2 (February 1, 1996): 728–35, https://doi.org/10.1210/jc.81.2.728.

Fiona C. Baker and Helen S. Driver, "Self-Reported Sleep across the Menstrual Cycle in Young, Healthy Women," *Journal of Psychosomatic Research* 56, no. 2 (February 2004): 239–43, https://doi.org/10.1016/s0022-3999(03)00067-9.

Fiona C. Baker and Helen S. Driver, "Circadian Rhythms, Sleep, and the Menstrual Cycle," *Sleep Medicine* 8, no. 6 (September 2007): 613–22, https://doi.org/10.1016/j.sleep.2006.09.011.

Helen S. Driver, "Sleep in Women," *Journal of Psychosomatic Research* 40, no. 3 (March 1996): 227–30, https://doi.org/10.1016/0022-3999(96)00030-x.

55 Michele Bellesi et al., "Sleep Loss Promotes Astrocytic Phagocytosis and Microglial Activation in Mouse Cerebral Cortex," *The Journal of Neuroscience* 37, no. 21 (May 24, 2017): 5263–73, https://doi.org/10.1523/jneurosci.3981-16.2017.

56 Hans P.A. Van Dongen et al., "The Cumulative Cost of Additional Wakefulness: Dose-Response Effects on Neurobehavioral Functions and Sleep Physiology From Chronic Sleep Restriction and Total Sleep Deprivation," *Sleep* 26, no. 2 (March 2003): 117–26, https://doi.org/10.1093/sleep/26.2.117.

57 Andrew R. Mendelsohn and James W. Larrick, "Sleep Facilitates Clearance of Metabolites from the Brain: Glymphatic Function in Aging and Neurodegenerative Diseases," *Rejuvenation Research* 16, no. 6 (December 2013): 518–23, https://doi.org/10.1089/rej.2013.1530.

Nadia Aalling Jessen et al., "The Glymphatic System: A Beginner's Guide," *Neurochemical Research* 40, no. 12 (May 7, 2015): 2583–99, https://doi.org/10.1007/s11064-015-1581-6.

58 J. J. Iliff et al., "A Paravascular Pathway Facilitates CSF Flow Through the Brain Parenchyma and the Clearance of Interstitial Solutes, Including Amyloid," *Science Translational Medicine* 4, no. 147 (August 15, 2012), https://doi.org/10.1126/scitranslmed.3003748.

59 Robert Y. Moore, "Suprachiasmatic Nucleus in Sleep–Wake Regulation," *Sleep Medicine* 8 (December 2007): 27–33, https://doi.org/10.1016/j.sleep.2007.10.003.

60 Mariana G. Figueiro et al., "The Impact of Light from Computer Monitors on Melatonin Levels in College Students," *Neuro Endocrinol Lett* 32, no. 2 (2011): 158–63.

61 L. C. Ruddick-Collins et al., "The Big Breakfast Study: Chrono-Nutrition Influence on Energy Expenditure and Bodyweight," *Nutrition Bulletin* 43, no. 2 (May 8, 2018): 174–83, https://doi.org/10.1111/nbu.12323.

62 Joaquim A. Ribeiro and Ana M. Sebastião, "Caffeine and Adenosine," *Journal of Alzheimer's Disease* 20, no. s1 (April 14, 2010): S3–15, https://doi.org/10.3233/JAD-2010-1379.

63 Bernard E. Statland and Theodore J. Demas, "Serum Caffeine Half-Lives: Healthy Subjects vs. Patients Having Alcoholic Hepatic Disease," *American Journal of Clinical Pathology* 73, no. 3 (March 1, 1980): 390–93, https://doi.org/10.1093/ajcp/73.3.390.

64 Greg L. West et al., "Playing Super Mario 64 Increases Hippocampal Grey Matter in Older Adults," ed. Etsuro Ito, *PLOS ONE* 12, no. 12 (December 6, 2017), https://doi.org/10.1371/journal.pone.0187779.

65 Richard J. Haier et al., "MRI Assessment of Cortical Thickness and Functional Activity Changes in Adolescent Girls Following Three Months of Practice on a Visual-Spatial Task," *BMC Research Notes* 2, no. 1 (2009): 174, https://doi.org/10.1186/1756-0500-2-174.

66 Qian Cheng et al., "Predicting Transitions in Oxygen Saturation Using Phone Sensors," *Telemedicine and E-Health* 22, no. 2 (February 2016): 132–37, https://doi.org/10.1089/tmj.2015.0040.

Raul Garrido-Chamorro, "Desaturation Patterns Detected by Oximetry in a Large Population of Athletes," *Research Quarterly for Exercise and Sport* 80, no. 2 (2009), https://doi.org/10.5641/027013609X13087704028390.

67 Katarzyna Cierpka-Kmieć and Dagmara Hering, "Tachycardia: The Hidden Cardiovascular Risk Factor in Uncomplicated Arterial Hypertension," *Cardiology Journal* (February 25, 2019), https://www.doi.org/10.5603/cj.a2019.0021.

68 Elie Fiogbé, Verena de Vassimon-Barroso, and Anielle Cristhine de Medeiros Takahashi, "Exercise Training in Older Adults, What Effects on Muscle Oxygenation? A Systematic Review," *Archives of Gerontology and Geriatrics* 71 (July 2017): 89–98, https://doi.org/10.1016/j.archger.2017.03.001.

69 Richard P. Brown and Patricia L. Gerbarg, "Yoga Breathing, Meditation, and Longevity," *Annals of the New York Academy of Sciences* 1172, no. 1 (August 2009): 54–62, https://doi.org/10.1111/j.1749-6632.2009.04394.x.

Marcello Árias Dias Danucalov et al., "Cardiorespiratory and Metabolic Changes during Yoga Sessions: The Effects of Respiratory Exercises and Meditation Practices," *Applied Psychophysiology and Biofeedback* 33, no. 2 (March 4, 2008): 77–81, https://doi.org/10.1007/s10484-008-9053-2.

70 Ke-Tsung Han and Li-Wen Ruan, "Effects of Indoor Plants on Air Quality: A Systematic Review," *Environmental Science and Pollution Research* 27, no. 14 (March 13, 2020): 16019–51, https://doi.org/10.1007/s11356-020-08174-9.

Linjing Deng and Qihong Deng, "The Basic Roles of Indoor Plants in Human Health and Comfort," *Environmental Science and Pollution Research* 25, no. 36 (November 1, 2018): 36087–101, https://doi.org/10.1007/s11356-018-3554-1.

71 Sunghyon Kyeong et al., "Effects of Gratitude Meditation on Neural Network Functional Connectivity and Brain-Heart Coupling," *Scientific Reports* 7, no. 1 (July 11, 2017), https://doi.org/10.1038/s41598-017-05520-9.

Feng Kong et al., "Gratitude and the Brain: Trait Gratitude Mediates the Association between Structural Variations in the Medial Prefrontal Cortex and Life Satisfaction," *Emotion* 20, no. 6 (September 2020): 917–26, https://doi.org/10.1037/emo0000617.

Glenn R. Fox et al., "Neural Correlates of Gratitude," *Frontiers in Psychology* 6 (September 30, 2015), https://doi.org/10.3389/fpsyg.2015.01491.

72 Paul O'Callaghan et al., "Effects of Bone Damage on Creep Behaviours of Human
    Vertebral Trabeculae," *Bone* 106 (January 2018): 204–10, https://doi.org/10.1016/j.
    bone.2017.10.022.

    Jacques Abboud, Benjamin Rousseau, and Martin Descarreaux, "Trunk Proprioception
    Adaptations to Creep Deformation," *European Journal of Applied Physiology* 118, no. 1
    (November 8, 2017): 133–42, https://doi.org/10.1007/s00421-017-3754-2.

    Jacques Abboud, François Nougarou, and Martin Descarreaux, "Muscle Activity
    Adaptations to Spinal Tissue Creep in the Presence of Muscle Fatigue," ed. Francesco
    Cappello, *PLOS ONE* 11, no. 2 (February 11, 2016), https://doi.org/10.1371/journal.
    pone.0149076.

73 Deborah M. Kado, "Hyperkyphosis Predicts Mortality Independent of Vertebral
    Osteoporosis in Older Women," *Annals of Internal Medicine* 150, no. 10 (May 19, 2009): 681,
    https://doi.org/10.7326/0003-4819-150-10-200905190-00005.

74 P. Pelosi et al., "Pathophysiology of Prone Positioning in the Healthy Lung and in ALI/
    ARDS," *Minerva Anestesiologica* (April 2001): 238–47.

75 Helen E. O'Connell et al., "Anatomy of the Clitoris," *Journal of Urology* 174, no. 4 Part 1
    (October 2005): 1189–95, https://doi.org/10.1097/01.ju.0000173639.38898.cd.

76 Winnifred B. Cutler, Celso R. Garcia, and Abba M. Krieger, "Sexual Behavior
    Frequency and Menstrual Cycle Length in Mature Premenopausal Women,"
    Psychoneuroendocrinology 4, no. 4 (January 1979): 297–309, https://doi.
    org/10.1016/0306-4530(79)90014-3.

77 Benedetta Leuner, Erica R. Glasper, and Elizabeth Gould, "Sexual Experience Promotes
    Adult Neurogenesis in the Hippocampus Despite an Initial Elevation in Stress Hormones,"
    ed. Melissa Coleman, *PLoS ONE* 5, no. 7 (July 14, 2010), https://doi.org/10.1371/journal.
    pone.0011597.

    Navneet Magon and Sanjay Kalra, "The Orgasmic History of Oxytocin: Love, Lust, and
    Labor," *Indian Journal of Endocrinology and Metabolism* 15, no. 7 (2011): 156, https://doi.
    org/10.4103/2230-8210.84851.

78 B. Lu, G. Nagappan, and Y. Lu, "BDNF and Synaptic Plasticity, Cognitive Function, and
    Dysfunction," in *Neurotrophic Factors* (Berlin: Springer Berlin Heidelberg, 2014), 223–50,
    https://doi.org/10.1007/978-3-642-45106-5_9.

    S.D. Hewagalamulage et al., "Stress, Cortisol, and Obesity: A Role for Cortisol
    Responsiveness in Identifying Individuals Prone to Obesity," *Domestic Animal
    Endocrinology* 56 (July 2016): S112–20, https://doi.org/10.1016/j.domaniend.2016.03.004.

    Rainer H. Straub and Maurizio Cutolo, "Glucocorticoids and Chronic Inflammation,"
    Rheumatology 55, no. suppl 2 (November 17, 2016): ii6–14, https://doi.org/10.1093/
    rheumatology/kew348.

Joseph M. Andreano, Hamidreza Arjomandi, and Larry Cahill, "Menstrual Cycle Modulation of the Relationship between Cortisol and Long-Term Memory," *Psychoneuroendocrinology* 33, no. 6 (July 2008): 874–82, https://doi.org/10.1016/j.psyneuen.2008.03.009.

Mercedes Almela et al., "The Impact of Cortisol Reactivity to Acute Stress on Memory: Sex Differences in Middle-Aged People," *Stress* 14, no. 2 (October 31, 2010): 117–27, https://doi.org/10.3109/10253890.2010.514671.

79 Nana Chung, Jonghoon Park, and Kiwon Lim, "The Effects of Exercise and Cold Exposure on Mitochondrial Biogenesis in Skeletal Muscle and White Adipose Tissue," *Journal of Exercise Nutrition & Biochemistry* 21, no. 2 (June 30, 2017): 39–47, https://doi.org/10.20463/jenb.2017.0020.

Nikolai A. Shevchuk, "Adapted Cold Shower as a Potential Treatment for Depression," *Medical Hypotheses* 70, no. 5 (January 2008): 995–1001, https://doi.org/10.1016/j.mehy.2007.04.052.

Nikolai A. Shevchuk, "Possible Use of Repeated Cold Stress for Reducing Fatigue in Chronic Fatigue Syndrome: A Hypothesis," *Behavioral and Brain Functions* 3, no. 1 (2007): 55, https://doi.org/10.1186/1744-9081-3-55.

80 Moráis-Moreno García et al., "Influence of Water Intake and Balance on Body Composition in Healthy Young Adults from Spain," *Nutrients* 11, no. 8 (August 15, 2019): 1923, https://doi.org/10.3390/nu11081923.

81 Fiona McKiernan et al. "Thirst-Drinking, Hunger-Eating; Tight Coupling?" *Journal of the American Dietetic Association* 109, no. 3 (March 2009): 486–90, https://doi.org/10.1016/j.jada.2008.11.027.

82 Michael N. Sawka, Samuel N. Cheuvront, and Robert Carter III, "Human Water Needs," *Nutrition Reviews* 63, no. 6 (June 1, 2005): 30–39, https://doi.org/10.1301/nr.2005.jun.s30-s39.

83 Li Li Ji, Chounghun Kang, and Yong Zhang, "Exercise-Induced Hormesis and Skeletal Muscle Health," *Free Radical Biology and Medicine* 98 (September 2016): 113–22, https://doi.org/10.1016/j.freeradbiomed.2016.02.025.

Troy L. Merry and Michael Ristow, "Mitohormesis in Exercise Training," *Free Radical Biology and Medicine* 98 (September 2016): 123–30, https://doi.org/10.1016/j.freeradbiomed.2015.11.032.

Robert V. Musci, Karyn L. Hamilton, and Melissa A. Linden, "Exercise-Induced Mitohormesis for the Maintenance of Skeletal Muscle and Healthspan Extension," *Sports* 7, no. 7 (July 11, 2019): 170, https://doi.org/10.3390/sports7070170.

84 Cindy K. Barha et al., "Sex Differences in Exercise Efficacy to Improve Cognition: A Systematic Review and Meta-Analysis of Randomized Controlled Trials in Older Humans," *Frontiers in Neuroendocrinology* 46 (July 2017): 71–85, https://doi.org/10.1016/j.yfrne.2017.04.002.

Rui Nouchi et al., "Four Weeks of Combination Exercise Training Improved Executive Functions, Episodic Memory, and Processing Speed in Healthy Elderly People: Evidence from a Randomized Controlled Trial," *AGE* 36, no. 2 (September 25, 2013): 787–99, https://doi.org/10.1007/s11357-013-9588-x.

Patrick J. Smith et al., "Aerobic Exercise and Neurocognitive Performance: A Meta-Analytic Review of Randomized Controlled Trials," *Psychosomatic Medicine* 72, no. 3 (April 2010): 239–52, https://doi.org/10.1097/psy.0b013e3181d14633.

85   Michael J. Wheeler et al., "Distinct Effects of Acute Exercise and Breaks in Sitting on Working Memory and Executive Function in Older Adults: A Three-Arm, Randomised Cross-over Trial to Evaluate the Effects of Exercise with and without Breaks in Sitting on Cognition," *British Journal of Sports Medicine* 54, no. 13 (April 29, 2019): 776–81, https://doi.org/10.1136/bjsports-2018-100168.

86   Essi K. Ahokas et al., "Effects of Water Immersion Methods on Postexercise Recovery of Physical and Mental Performance," *Journal of Strength and Conditioning Research* 33, no. 6 (June 2019): 1488–95, https://doi.org/10.1519/jsc.0000000000003134.

87   Yun-Hee Youm et al., "The Ketone Metabolite β-Hydroxybutyrate Blocks NLRP3 Inflammasome–Mediated Inflammatory Disease," *Nature Medicine* 21, no. 3 (February 16, 2015): 263–69, https://doi.org/10.1038/nm.3804.

88   A. A. Gibson et al., "Do Ketogenic Diets Really Suppress Appetite? A Systematic Review and Meta-Analysis," *Obesity Reviews* 16, no. 1 (November 17, 2014): 64–76, https://doi.org/10.1111/obr.12230.

P. Sumithran et al., "Ketosis and Appetite-Mediating Nutrients and Hormones after Weight Loss," *European Journal of Clinical Nutrition* 67, no. 7 (May 1, 2013): 759–64, https://doi.org/10.1038/ejcn.2013.90.

89   Lindsey B. Gano, Manisha Patel, and Jong M. Rho, "Ketogenic Diets, Mitochondria, and Neurological Diseases," *Journal of Lipid Research* 55, no. 11 (May 20, 2014): 2211–28, https://doi.org/10.1194/jlr.r048975.

Silvia Vidali et al., "Mitochondria: The Ketogenic Diet—A Metabolism-Based Therapy," *The International Journal of Biochemistry & Cell Biology* 63 (June 2015): 55–59, https://doi.org/10.1016/j.biocel.2015.01.022.

90   Mahshid Dehghan, Andrew Mente, and Salim Yusuf, "Associations of Fats and Carbohydrates with Cardiovascular Disease and Mortality—PURE and Simple?—Authors' Reply," *The Lancet* 391, no. 10131 (April 2018): 1681–82, https://doi.org/10.1016/s0140-6736(18)30774-8.

Anna E. Arthur et al., "Higher Carbohydrate Intake Is Associated with Increased Risk of All-Cause and Disease-Specific Mortality in Head and Neck Cancer Patients: Results from a Prospective Cohort Study," *International Journal of Cancer* 143, no. 5 (April 17, 2018): 1105–13, https://doi.org/10.1002/ijc.31413.

91   Maria L. Fernandez, "Rethinking Dietary Cholesterol," *Current Opinion in Clinical Nutrition and Metabolic Care* 15, no. 2 (March 2012): 117–21, https://doi.org/10.1097/mco.0b013e32834d2259.

Donald J. McNamara, "Dietary Cholesterol, Heart Disease Risk and Cognitive Dissonance," *Proceedings of the Nutrition Society* 73, no. 2 (January 9, 2014): 161–66, https://doi.org/10.1017/s0029665113003844.

Mitchell M. Kanter et al., "Exploring the Factors That Affect Blood Cholesterol and Heart Disease Risk: Is Dietary Cholesterol as Bad for You as History Leads Us to Believe?" *Advances in Nutrition* 3, no. 5 (September 1, 2012): 711–17, https://doi.org/10.3945/an.111.001321.

Hsuan-Ping Lin et al., "Dietary Cholesterol, Lipid Levels, and Cardiovascular Risk among Adults with Diabetes or Impaired Fasting Glucose in the Framingham Offspring Study," *Nutrients* 10, no. 6 (June 14, 2018): 770, https://doi.org/10.3390/nu10060770.

Siyouneh Baghdasarian et al., "Dietary Cholesterol Intake Is Not Associated with Risk of Type 2 Diabetes in the Framingham Offspring Study," *Nutrients* 10, no. 6 (May 24, 2018): 665, https://doi.org/10.3390/nu10060665.

92   Stephanie Seneff, Glyn Wainwright, and Luca Mascitelli, "Is the Metabolic Syndrome Caused by a High Fructose, and Relatively Low Fat, Low Cholesterol Diet?" *Archives of Medical Science* 1 (2011): 8–20, https://doi.org/10.5114/aoms.2011.20598.

93   Halfdan Petursson et al., "Is the Use of Cholesterol in Mortality Risk Algorithms in Clinical Guidelines Valid? Ten Years Prospective Data from the Norwegian HUNT 2 Study," *Journal of Evaluation in Clinical Practice* 18, no. 1 (September 25, 2011): 159–68, https://doi.org/10.1111/j.1365-2753.2011.01767.x.

94   Graziano Onder et al., "Serum Cholesterol Levels and In-Hospital Mortality in the Elderly," *The American Journal of Medicine* 115, no. 4 (September 2003): 265–71, https://doi.org/10.1016/s0002-9343(03)00354-1.

95   Joseph A. Boscarino, Porat M. Erlich, and Stuart N. Hoffman, "Low Serum Cholesterol and External-Cause Mortality: Potential Implications for Research and Surveillance," *Journal of Psychiatric Research* 43, no. 9 (June 2009): 848–54, https://doi.org/10.1016/j.jpsychires.2008.11.007.

96   R.E. Morgan et al., "Plasma Cholesterol and Depressive Symptoms in Older Men," *The Lancet* 341, no. 8837 (January 1993): 75–79, https://doi.org/10.1016/0140-6736(93)92556-9.

97   M. M. Mielke et al., "High Total Cholesterol Levels in Late Life Associated with a Reduced Risk of Dementia," *Neurology* 64, no. 10 (April 20, 2005): 1689–95, https://doi.org/10.1212/01.wnl.0000161870.78572.a5.

98   Stephanie Seneff, Glyn Wainwright, and Luca Mascitelli, "Nutrition and Alzheimer's Disease: The Detrimental Role of a High Carbohydrate Diet," *European Journal of Internal Medicine* 22, no. 2 (April 2011): 134–40, https://doi.org/10.1016/j.ejim.2010.12.017.

99   Tanja V. Maier et al., "Impact of Dietary Resistant Starch on the Human Gut Microbiome, Metaproteome, and Metabolome," ed. Mary Ann Moran, *MBio* 8, no. 5 (October 17, 2017), https://doi.org/10.1128/mbio.01343-17.

100 Knud Erik Bach Knudsen et al., "Impact of Diet-Modulated Butyrate Production on Intestinal Barrier Function and Inflammation," *Nutrients* 10, no. 10 (October 13, 2018): 1499, https://doi.org/10.3390/nu10101499.

101 Qinghui Mu et al., "Leaky Gut As a Danger Signal for Autoimmune Diseases," *Frontiers in Immunology* 8 (May 23, 2017), https://doi.org/10.3389/fimmu.2017.00598.

Hiroshi Fukui, "Role of Gut Dysbiosis in Liver Diseases: What Have We Learned So Far?" *Diseases* 7, no. 4 (November 12, 2019): 58, https://doi.org/10.3390/diseases7040058.

Seungbum Kim et al., "Imbalance of Gut Microbiome and Intestinal Epithelial Barrier Dysfunction in Patients with High Blood Pressure," *Clinical Science* 132, no. 6 (March 30, 2018): 701–18, https://doi.org/10.1042/cs20180087.

102 Megan W. Bourassa et al., "Butyrate, Neuroepigenetics and the Gut Microbiome: Can a High Fiber Diet Improve Brain Health?" *Neuroscience Letters* 625 (June 2016): 56–63, https://doi.org/10.1016/j.neulet.2016.02.009.

103 Tyler A. Churchward-Venne et al., "Supplementation of a Suboptimal Protein Dose with Leucine or Essential Amino Acids: Effects on Myofibrillar Protein Synthesis at Rest and Following Resistance Exercise in Men," *The Journal of Physiology* 590, no. 11 (April 24, 2012): 2751–65, https://doi.org/10.1113/jphysiol.2012.228833.

Daniel R. Moore, "Maximizing Post-Exercise Anabolism: The Case for Relative Protein Intakes," *Frontiers in Nutrition* 6 (September 10, 2019), https://doi.org/10.3389/fnut.2019.00147.

Elfego Galvan et al., "Protecting Skeletal Muscle with Protein and Amino Acid during Periods of Disuse," *Nutrients* 8, no. 7 (July 1, 2016): 404, https://doi.org/10.3390/nu8070404.

Håvard Hamarsland et al., "Native Whey Protein with High Levels of Leucine Results in Similar Post-Exercise Muscular Anabolic Responses as Regular Whey Protein: A Randomized Controlled Trial," *Journal of the International Society of Sports Nutrition* 14, no. 1 (November 21, 2017), https://doi.org/10.1186/s12970-017-0202-y.

Madonna M. Mamerow et al., "Dietary Protein Distribution Positively Influences 24-h Muscle Protein Synthesis in Healthy Adults," *The Journal of Nutrition* 144, no. 6 (January 29, 2014): 876–80, https://doi.org/10.3945/jn.113.185280.

104 Jürgen Bauer et al., "Evidence-Based Recommendations for Optimal Dietary Protein Intake in Older People: A Position Paper From the PROT-AGE Study Group," *Journal of the American Medical Directors Association* 14, no. 8 (August 2013): 542–59, https://doi.org/10.1016/j.jamda.2013.05.021.

105 Nathan Hodson et al., "Molecular Regulation of Human Skeletal Muscle Protein Synthesis in Response to Exercise and Nutrients: A Compass for Overcoming Age-Related Anabolic Resistance," *American Journal of Physiology-Cell Physiology* 317, no. 6 (December 1, 2019): C1061–78, https://doi.org/10.1152/ajpcell.00209.2019.

Brandon J. Shad, Janice L. Thompson, and Leigh Breen, "Does the Muscle Protein Synthetic Response to Exercise and Amino Acid-Based Nutrition Diminish with Advancing Age? A Systematic Review," *American Journal of Physiology-Endocrinology and Metabolism* 311, no. 5 (November 1, 2016): E803–17, https://doi.org/10.1152/ajpendo.00213.2016.

106 Junaidah B. Barnett et al., "Plasma Lipid and Lipoprotein Levels during the Follicular and Luteal Phases of the Menstrual Cycle," *The Journal of Clinical Endocrinology & Metabolism* 89, no. 2 (February 2004): 776–82, https://doi.org/10.1210/jc.2003-030506.

C. F. Draper et al., "Menstrual Cycle Rhythmicity: Metabolic Patterns in Healthy Women," *Scientific Reports* 8, no. 1 (October 1, 2018), https://doi.org/10.1038/s41598-018-32647-0.

Oleg Varlamov, Cynthia L. Bethea, and Charles T. Roberts, "Sex-Specific Differences in Lipid and Glucose Metabolism," *Frontiers in Endocrinology* 5 (January 19, 2015), https://doi.org/10.3389/fendo.2014.00241.

107 Bronwen Martin et al., "Sex-Dependent Metabolic, Neuroendocrine, and Cognitive Responses to Dietary Energy Restriction and Excess," *Endocrinology* 148, no. 9 (September 2007): 4318–33, https://doi.org/10.1210/en.2007-0161.

Bronwen Martin et al., "Conserved and Differential Effects of Dietary Energy Intake on the Hippocampal Transcriptomes of Females and Males," ed. Richard Mayeux, *PLoS ONE* 3, no. 6 (June 11, 2008), https://doi.org/10.1371/journal.pone.0002398.

108 Bronwen Martin et al., "Sex-Dependent Metabolic, Neuroendocrine, and Cognitive Responses to Dietary Energy Restriction and Excess," *Endocrinology* 148, no. 9 (September 2007): 4318–33, https://doi.org/10.1210/en.2007-0161.

109 Valter D. Longo and Satchidananda Panda, "Fasting, Circadian Rhythms, and Time-Restricted Feeding in Healthy Lifespan," *Cell Metabolism* 23, no. 6 (June 2016): 1048–59, https://doi.org/10.1016/j.cmet.2016.06.001.

110 Claudia Günther et al., "Apoptosis, Necrosis and Necroptosis: Cell Death Regulation in the Intestinal Epithelium," *Gut* 62, no. 7 (June 11, 2012): 1062–71, https://doi.org/10.1136/gutjnl-2011-301364.

111 H. Papaconstantinou, "Prevention of Mucosal Atrophy: Role of Glutamine and Caspases in Apoptosis in Intestinal Epithelial Cells," *Journal of Gastrointestinal Surgery* 4, no. 4 (August 2000): 416–23, https://doi.org/10.1016/s1091-255x(00)80022-0.

112 Yves Henrotin, Cécile Lambert, and Pascal Richette, "Importance of Synovitis in Osteoarthritis: Evidence for the Use of Glycosaminoglycans against Synovial Inflammation," *Seminars in Arthritis and Rheumatism* 43, no. 5 (April 2014): 579–87, https://doi.org/10.1016/j.semarthrit.2013.10.005.

113 Yinhua Ni et al., "Late-Night Eating-Induced Physiological Dysregulation and Circadian Misalignment Are Accompanied by Microbial Dysbiosis," *Molecular Nutrition & Food Research* 63, no. 24 (November 6, 2019), https://doi.org/10.1002/mnfr.201900867.

Megumi Hatori et al., "Time-Restricted Feeding without Reducing Caloric Intake Prevents Metabolic Diseases in Mice Fed a High-Fat Diet," *Cell Metabolism* 15, no. 6 (June 2012): 848–60, https://doi.org/10.1016/j.cmet.2012.04.019.

114 Jennifer A. Mohawk, Carla B. Green, and Joseph S. Takahashi, "Central and Peripheral Circadian Clocks in Mammals," *Annual Review of Neuroscience* 35, no. 1 (July 21, 2012): 445–62, https://doi.org/10.1146/annurev-neuro-060909-153128.

115 Catherine R. Marinac et al., "Prolonged Nightly Fasting and Breast Cancer Prognosis," *JAMA Oncology* 2, no. 8 (August 1, 2016): 1049, https://doi.org/10.1001/jamaoncol.2016.0164.

116 Catherine R. Marinac et al., "Prolonged Nightly Fasting and Breast Cancer Prognosis," *JAMA Oncology* 2, no. 8 (August 1, 2016): 1049, https://doi.org/10.1001/jamaoncol.2016.0164.

117 Kelsey Gabel et al., "Effects of 8-Hour Time Restricted Feeding on Body Weight and Metabolic Disease Risk Factors in Obese Adults: A Pilot Study," *JB. Nutrition and Healthy Aging* 4, no. 4 (June 15, 2018): 345–53, https://doi.org/10.3233/NHA-170036.

118 Shu Wang et al., "Novel Insights of Dietary Polyphenols and Obesity," *The Journal of Nutritional Biochemistry* 25, no. 1 (January 2014): 1–18, https://doi.org/10.1016/j.jnutbio.2013.09.001.

119 Michael F. Holick, "The Vitamin D Deficiency Pandemic: Approaches for Diagnosis, Treatment and Prevention," *Reviews in Endocrine and Metabolic Disorders* 18, no. 2 (May 17, 2017): 153–65, https://doi.org/10.1007/s11154-017-9424-1.

120 Caitlin Mason et al., "Vitamin D3 Supplementation during Weight Loss: A Double-Blind Randomized Controlled Trial," *The American Journal of Clinical Nutrition* 99, no. 5 (March 12, 2014): 1015–25, https://doi.org/10.3945/ajcn.113.073734.

Heike A. Bischoff-Ferrari et al., "Prevention of Nonvertebral Fractures With Oral Vitamin D and Dose Dependency," *Archives of Internal Medicine* 169, no. 6 (March 23, 2009): 551, https://doi.org/10.1001/archinternmed.2008.600.

Harald Dobnig, "Independent Association of Low Serum 25-Hydroxyvitamin D and 1,25-Dihydroxyvitamin D Levels With All-Cause and Cardiovascular Mortality," *Archives of Internal Medicine* 168, no. 12 (June 23, 2008): 1340, https://doi.org/10.1001/archinte.168.12.1340.

121 Krasimir Kostov and Lyudmila Halacheva, "Role of Magnesium Deficiency in Promoting Atherosclerosis, Endothelial Dysfunction, and Arterial Stiffening as Risk Factors for Hypertension," *International Journal of Molecular Sciences* 19, no. 6 (June 11, 2018): 1724, https://doi.org/10.3390/ijms19061724.

M. Rodriguez-Moran and F. Guerrero-Romero, "Oral Magnesium Supplementation Improves Insulin Sensitivity and Metabolic Control in Type 2 Diabetic Subjects: A Randomized Double-Blind Controlled Trial," *Diabetes Care* 26, no. 4 (April 1, 2003): 1147–52, https://doi.org/10.2337/diacare.26.4.1147.

Elham Ebrahimi et al., "Effects of Magnesium and Vitamin B6 on the Severity of Premenstrual Syndrome Symptoms," *Journal of Caring Sciences* 1, no. 4 (2012): 183–189, https://doi.org/10.5681/JCS.2012.026.

122 Artemis Simopoulos, "An Increase in the Omega-6/Omega-3 Fatty Acid Ratio Increases the Risk for Obesity," *Nutrients* 8, no. 3 (March 2, 2016): 128, https://doi.org/10.3390/nu8030128.

123 A.P. Simopoulos, "The Importance of the Ratio of Omega-6/Omega-3 Essential Fatty Acids," *Biomedicine & Pharmacotherapy* 56, no. 8 (October 2002): 365–79, https://doi.org/10.1016/s0753-3322(02)00253-6.

124 Melissa Y. Wei and Terry A. Jacobson, "Effects of Eicosapentaenoic Acid Versus Docosahexaenoic Acid on Serum Lipids: A Systematic Review and Meta-Analysis," *Current Atherosclerosis Reports* 13, no. 6 (October 6, 2011): 474–83, https://doi.org/10.1007/s11883-011-0210-3.

Jan Oscarsson and Eva Hurt-Camejo, "Omega-3 Fatty Acids Eicosapentaenoic Acid and Docosahexaenoic Acid and Their Mechanisms of Action on Apolipoprotein B-Containing Lipoproteins in Humans: A Review," *Lipids in Health and Disease* 16, no. 1 (August 10, 2017), https://doi.org/10.1186/s12944-017-0541-3.

James Backes et al., "The Clinical Relevance of Omega-3 Fatty Acids in the Management of Hypertriglyceridemia," *Lipids in Health and Disease* 15, no. 1 (July 22, 2016), https://doi.org/10.1186/s12944-016-0286-4.

125 Alec Coppen and Christina Bolander-Gouaille, "Treatment of Depression: Time to Consider Folic Acid and Vitamin B12," *Journal of Psychopharmacology* 19, no. 1 (January 2005): 59–65, https://doi.org/10.1177/0269881105048899.

Toshiko Takahashi-Iñiguez et al., "Role of Vitamin B12 on Methylmalonyl-CoA Mutase Activity," *Journal of Zhejiang University Science* B 13, no. 6 (June 2012): 423–37, https://doi.org/10.1631/jzus.b1100329.

Salah E. Gariballa, Sarah J. Forster, and Hilary J. Powers, "Effects of Mixed Dietary Supplements on Total Plasma Homocysteine Concentrations (THcy): A Randomized, Double-Blind, Placebo-Controlled Trial," *International Journal for Vitamin and Nutrition Research* 82, no. 4 (August 1, 2012): 260–66, https://doi.org/10.1024/0300-9831/a000118.

Alba Rocco et al., "Vitamin B12supplementation Improves Rates of Sustained Viral Response in Patients Chronically Infected with Hepatitis C Virus," *Gut* 62, no. 5 (July 17, 2012): 766–73, https://doi.org/10.1136/gutjnl-2012-302344.

126 Hui Dong et al., "Berberine in the Treatment of Type 2 Diabetes Mellitus: A Systemic Review and Meta-Analysis," *Evidence-Based Complementary and Alternative Medicine* 2012 (2012): 1–12, https://doi.org/10.1155/2012/591654.

N. Turner et al., "Berberine and Its More Biologically Available Derivative, Dihydroberberine, Inhibit Mitochondrial Respiratory Complex I: A Mechanism for the Action of Berberine to Activate AMP-Activated Protein Kinase and Improve Insulin Action," *Diabetes* 57, no. 5 (February 19, 2008): 1414–18, https://doi.org/10.2337/db07-1552.

Francesco Di Pierro et al., "Pilot Study on the Additive Effects of Berberine and Oral Type 2 Diabetes Agents for Patients with Suboptimal Glycemic Control," *Diabetes, Metabolic Syndrome and Obesity* 5 (July 2012): 213–217, https://doi.org/10.2147/dmso.s33718.

127 Woo Sik Kim et al., "Berberine Improves Lipid Dysregulation in Obesity by Controlling Central and Peripheral AMPK Activity," *American Journal of Physiology-Endocrinology and Metabolism* 296, no. 4 (April 2009): E812–19, https://doi.org/10.1152/ajpendo.90710.2008.

Zahra Ilyas et al., "The Effect of Berberine on Weight Loss in Order to Prevent Obesity: A Systematic Review," *Biomedicine & Pharmacotherapy* 127 (July 2020), https://doi.org/10.1016/j.biopha.2020.110137.

Zhiguo Zhang et al., "Berberine Activates Thermogenesis in White and Brown Adipose Tissue," *Nature Communications* 5, no. 1 (November 25, 2014), https://doi.org/10.1038/ncomms6493.

M. Rondanelli et al., "Polycystic Ovary Syndrome Management: A Review of the Possible Amazing Role of Berberine," *Archives of Gynecology and Obstetrics* 301, no. 1 (January 2020): 53–60, https://doi.org/10.1007/s00404-020-05450-4.

Li Zhao et al., "Berberine Improves Glucogenesis and Lipid Metabolism in Nonalcoholic Fatty Liver Disease," *BMC Endocrine Disorders* 17, no. 1 (February 28, 2017), https://doi.org/10.1186/s12902-017-0165-7.

128 E. Proksch et al., "Oral Supplementation of Specific Collagen Peptides Has Beneficial Effects on Human Skin Physiology: A Double-Blind, Placebo-Controlled Study," *Skin Pharmacology and Physiology* 27, no. 1 (2014): 47–55, https://doi.org/10.1159/000351376.

129 Alfonso E. Bello and Steffen Oesser, "Collagen Hydrolysate for the Treatment of Osteoarthritis and Other Joint Disorders: A Review of the Literature," *Current Medical Research and Opinion* 22, no. 11 (October 10, 2006): 2221–32, https://doi.org/10.1185/030079906x148373.

Roland W. Moskowitz, "Role of Collagen Hydrolysate in Bone and Joint Disease," *Seminars in Arthritis and Rheumatism* 30, no. 2 (October 2000): 87–99, https://doi.org/10.1053/sarh.2000.9622.

130 Reza Tabrizi et al., "The Effects of Curcumin-Containing Supplements on Biomarkers of Inflammation and Oxidative Stress: A Systematic Review and Meta-Analysis of Randomized Controlled Trials," *Phytotherapy Research* 33, no. 2 (November 7, 2018): 253–62, https://doi.org/10.1002/ptr.6226.

131 Qin Xiang Ng et al., "Clinical Use of Curcumin in Depression: A Meta-Analysis," *Journal of the American Medical Directors Association* 18, no. 6 (June 2017): 503–8, https://doi.org/10.1016/j.jamda.2016.12.071.

Jian Wu, Ming Lv, and Yixin Zhou, "Efficacy and Side Effect of Curcumin for the Treatment of Osteoarthritis: A Meta-Analysis of Randomized Control Trials," *Pakistan Journal of Pharmaceutical Sciences* 32, no. 1 (January 2019): 43–51, https://applications.emro.who.int/imemrf/Pak_J_Pharm_Sci/Pak_J_Pharm_Sci_2019_32_1_43_51.pdf.

132 Siri Kvam et al., "Exercise as a Treatment for Depression: A Meta-Analysis," *Journal of Affective Disorders* 202 (September 2016): 67–86, https://doi.org/10.1016/j.jad.2016.03.063.

133 Brendon Stubbs et al., "An Examination of the Anxiolytic Effects of Exercise for People with Anxiety and Stress-Related Disorders: A Meta-Analysis," *Psychiatry Research* 249 (March 2017): 102–8, https://doi.org/10.1016/j.psychres.2016.12.020.

Lindsey Anderson et al., "Exercise-Based Cardiac Rehabilitation for Coronary Heart Disease," *Cochrane Database of Systematic Reviews* 1 (January 5, 2016): 1465–1858, https://doi.org/10.1002/14651858.cd001800.pub3.

Sue Vaughan et al., "The Effects of Multimodal Exercise on Cognitive and Physical Functioning and Brain-Derived Neurotrophic Factor in Older Women: A Randomised Controlled Trial," *Age and Ageing* 43, no. 5 (February 18, 2014): 623–29, https://doi.org/10.1093/ageing/afu010.

Paloma Carroquino-Garcia et al., "Therapeutic Exercise in the Treatment of Primary Dysmenorrhea: A Systematic Review and Meta-Analysis," *Physical Therapy* 99, no. 10 (October 2019): 1371–80, https://doi.org/10.1093/ptj/pzz101.

J. L. Benham et al., "Role of Exercise Training in Polycystic Ovary Syndrome: A Systematic Review and Meta-Analysis," *Clinical Obesity* 8, no. 4 (June 12, 2018): 275–84, https://doi.org/10.1111/cob.12258.

134 Chih-Chin Lai et al., "Effects of Resistance Training, Endurance Training and Whole-Body Vibration on Lean Body Mass, Muscle Strength and Physical Performance in Older People: A Systematic Review and Network Meta-Analysis," *Age and Ageing* 47, no. 3 (February 17, 2018): 367–73, https://doi.org/10.1093/ageing/afy009.

135 Kyoung Min Kim et al., "Longitudinal Changes in Muscle Mass and Strength, and Bone Mass in Older Adults: Gender-Specific Associations Between Muscle and Bone Losses," *The Journals of Gerontology*: Series A 73, no. 8 (October 8, 2017): 1062–69, https://doi.org/10.1093/gerona/glx188.

Natalie Goldring, Jonathan D. Wiles, and Damian Coleman, "The Effects of Isometric Wall Squat Exercise on Heart Rate and Blood Pressure in a Normotensive Population," *Journal of Sports Sciences* 32, no. 2 (July 24, 2013): 129–36, https://doi.org/10.1080/02640414.2013.809471.

136 T. O. Smith et al., "Factors Predicting Incidence of Post-Operative Delirium in Older People Following Hip Fracture Surgery: A Systematic Review and Meta-Analysis," *International Journal of Geriatric Psychiatry* 32, no. 4 (January 17, 2017): 386–96, https://doi.org/10.1002/gps.4655.

137 Nkechinyere Chidi-Ogbolu and Keith Baar, "Effect of Estrogen on Musculoskeletal Performance and Injury Risk," *Frontiers in Physiology* 9 (January 15, 2019), https://doi.org/10.3389/fphys.2018.01834.

138 Gregory D. Myer et al., "The Effects of Generalized Joint Laxity on Risk of Anterior Cruciate Ligament Injury in Young Female Athletes," *The American Journal of Sports Medicine* 36, no. 6 (June 2008): 1073–80, https://doi.org/10.1177/0363546507313572.

Sang-Kyoon Park et al., "Changing Hormone Levels during the Menstrual Cycle Affect Knee Laxity and Stiffness in Healthy Female Subjects," *The American Journal of Sports Medicine* 37, no. 3 (March 2009): 588–98, https://doi.org/10.1177/0363546508326713.

139 Brad J. Schoenfeld, Dan Ogborn, and James W. Krieger, "Dose-Response Relationship between Weekly Resistance Training Volume and Increases in Muscle Mass: A Systematic Review and Meta-Analysis," *Journal of Sports Sciences* 35, no. 11 (July 19, 2016): 1073–82, https://doi.org/10.1080/02640414.2016.1210197.

Made in the USA
Coppell, TX
30 January 2022